Dr Nadya Coates has a PhD in biochemistry and is a qualified doctor of medicine. She is director and founder of the Springhill Centre.

Norman Jollyman is a practising homeopath.

A MATTER OF LIFE

The Springhill Centre's holistic approach to caring and healing

**NADYA COATES, M.D.
AND NORMAN JOLLYMAN**

An OPTIMA book

© Dr Nadya Coates and Norman Jollyman, 1990

First published in 1990 by
Macdonald Optima, a division of
Macdonald & Co. (Publishers) Ltd

A member of Maxwell Macmillan Pergamon Publishing Corporation

British Library Cataloguing in Publication Data
Coates, Nadya
    A Matter of Life
    1. Man. Health. Improvement
    I. Title   II. Jollyman, N.W.
    613

    ISBN 0-356-19107-9

Macdonald & Co. (Publishers) Ltd
Orbit House
1 New Fetter Lane
London EC4A 1AR

Typeset in Ehrhard by Leaper & Gard Ltd, Bristol

Printed and bound in Great Britain by
The Guernsey Press Co. Ltd., Guernsey, Channel Islands.

CONTENTS

PREFACE

This book has been written in response to a cry from the heart that comes from everyone diagnosed as having cancer or any other life-threatening or degenerative disease. 'What can I do to help myself?'

An awareness of the importance of taking responsibility for one's own health is a fundamental message of the Springhill Centre. It is in fact an integral part of the curative process.

This book is intended to be a 'self-help' manual to aid individuals who can best help themselves by understanding how to maintain a healthy immune system and healthier attitudes to life.

It is clear from the present state of knowledge of how immune responses operate, that an individual has a certain amount of responsibility for his or her breakdown through faulty lifestyle, poor nutrition and, often, from an inability to handle stress. Ways of sidetracking the ill effects of stress, and the steps necessary to maintain health through efficient immune responses, are suggested. Appropriate knowledge is indeed life-enhancing. We have attempted to provide the scientific background to the important physical processes involved in maintaining health in as simple a manner as possible, so that everyone concerned – and that must include carers, family and friends of the patient too – can understand the reasons for a certain lifestyle or procedures to be adopted once illness takes hold.

Springhill is, above all, a caring milieu with a spirit all of its own, where the isolation and the threatening atmosphere of many an institutional setting, is, by contrast, replaced with the cheerful atmosphere of a community, where problems are discussed openly and shared with a large number of truly dedicated co-workers, many of whom are volunteers, whose commitment to the Centre is complete and unstinting.

The philosophy of care which underpins the therapeutic endeavours of Springhill has its foundation in the teachings of the Austrian philosopher Rudolf Steiner and his later followers who diversified into more specialised areas of health care and education.

It is useful to consider the role of doctors, healers or carers as privileged friends of the sick. Ever since the Springhill Centre opened its doors to patients, their families and friends, a number of individuals whose lives have been dedicated to the healing ministry have been part of the daily round of caring and sharing. In the true spirit of fellowship every one comes in order to instil the atmosphere of the place with the greater faith, hope, peace and unconditional love.

Some use healing touch, others the healing properties of essential oils, others music, art, sounds or colour; some care for the gardens or cook wonderful meals; others provide the wisdom of many years of life experience and utter the words that soothe and heal. What is a healer but a friend whose touch, whose words, whose deeds are but an expression of the symphony of a universal order which knows no frontiers?

The Springhill Centre owes an enormous debt of gratitude to all who, in the spirit of healing, selflessly and unasssumingly have so often sacrificed themselves and their time in offering continuous care and support to those in need.

For them all, only the spirit of the most high can encompass the nature of the truth, the beauty and the goodness that they have come to embody as the spirit of Springhill.

In January 1990, Springhill opened a special unit in a converted farm building in which programmes of Conductive Education are carried out so that children and adults who suffer from severely disabling motor disorders can benefit from this all-embracing approach to their disease.

Conductive Education involves an intensive course of physical and mental stimulation aimed at teaching children and adults with motor disorders how to overcome problems of movement and control so that they can live a more normal life with approximately the same degree of independence as an able-bodied person of the same age.

Conductive Education was developed by Professor András Petö at the Petö Institute in Budapest. Springhill is one of the few places in England where Conductive Education in its complete form is offered to people with diseases such as cerebral palsy, spina bifida, Parkinson's disease, Frederich's ataxia, multiple sclerosis, spinal injuries, strokes and motor neurone disease.

The unit at Springhill will not only cater as a provision for the local community but will grow as a residential facility for those coming from further afield.

A recognition of an unending debt of gratitude is acknowledged to: Prof Alejandro Leloir, Argentinian endocrinologist and Nobel prize-winner; Prof Italo Nunciatt, Argentinian professor of anaesthetics at the University of Buenos Aires; Prof Thomas Fritz Gravitz, Austrian professor of neurophysiology; Prof András Petö, Hungarian professor of neurophysiology, pedagogue and initiator of the system of Conductive Education; Dr Gregorio Marañon, Spanish physician and psychiatrist;

Dr Carl Jung, Swiss psychiatrist and leading thinker and innovator in understanding the human psyche; Mr Francis Edmunds, Russian-born Jewish pedagogue and founder of Emerson College of Further Education following Rudolf Steiner's teachings; Dr Broder von Loue, medical director and founder-member of the Oeschellbrun Hospital for internal medicine and cancer care near Pforzheim in West Germany; Dr Moshe Feldenkrais, Russian-Jewish physiotherapist and scientist in nuclear physics; and also to the writings of Dr Rudolf Steiner, Austrian philosopher and mystic, Dr Karl Konig, founder of the Camphill villages, and Dr Jean Vanier, L'Arche communities founder.

This book could not have been compiled without the assistance of many people and we would like to acknowledge gratefully the help we have received from the following: Grace McIntosh for her patient help in taping the weekly talks given to patients and friends on which much of the book is based; Victor Newby for some fundamental information about the immune system; Linda Zundel for her instruction in chirophonetics; Carrie Jost for help in clarifying the meridian massages; Dr Francis Fox for painstakingly reviewing the literature on fungemia, candidiasis and mycotoxin hazards to health; Barry Halliwell and John Gutteridge for their work on free radicals in medicine and biology.

What begins as a journey of transformation for many in a therapeutic setting such as Springhill enables each person to find others who are mirrors for life's perspectives akin to their own individuality.

Nadya Coates and Norman Jollyman

I
INTRODUCTION

There can scarcely be a more emotive and frightening subject than cancer, yet with the right mental attitude, together with changes in lifestyle, much can be done by the individual to prevent, control or overcome cancer, to the point where it ceases to be life-threatening.

Springhill is a rehabilitation and continuous care centre near Aylesbury, Bucks. This is a statement of fact which cannot give any indication of the exciting potential of the Centre for pointing the way, by using holistic methods allied to conventional treatments, in cancer and other degenerative diseases. It is, perhaps more importantly, committed to the education of patients and their families in the prevention of malignant or degenerative illness and to increasing the quality of life of those on the 'conveyor belt' of a chronic ailment.

The spirit of Springhill is something quite intangible – yet it is felt immediately by anyone who visits the Centre. There is an immediate feeling of warmth and welcome, an unhurried willingness to listen, a feeling of being someone special and not just a number, a feeling of hope and encouragement – and the curative process has then already begun. When first diagnosed as having cancer, for instance, people are shattered and it is at that point that Springhill can assist, in conjunction with medics, hospitals and relations, to ease the load. It provides an extension of care that is not possible in hospitals, not an alternative method of care. It is an expression of TLC (tender loving care) and is intended to give the patients an opportunity to reappraise their own lives and lifestyles, and, in an atmosphere of peace and harmony, to work out what they want out of life and how to move towards it.

THE IMMUNE SYSTEM

We live in a 'sea' of carcinogens, constantly at risk from roaming cancer cells. There are potential cancer cells in everyone but the antigens on the cells' surface alert the T cells of our immune system, which then start to destroy the cancer cells. Sometimes, however, some cells evade detection and proliferate. Whether we succumb to them or not will depend on the strength of our immune system as a whole.

Everyone is regularly exposed to disease, yet not everyone contracts it; for example, the incidence of lung cancer is higher in smokers than non-smokers, but not all heavy smokers get cancer. This is because the immune system is designed to attack and destroy foreign substances routinely, including cancerous cells. The actual presence of cancerous cells does not automatically mean cancer will develop – this happens only when there is a suppression of the immune system, the body's normal defence. So the main question is 'What has suddenly stopped the immune system from doing its job?'

It may be found that faulty nutrition in an individual may have weakened their immune system. Or it may be that some external environmental influences have overloaded their capacity to protect themselves. It may well be emotional stress or a family crisis or bereavement of a loved one which has proved to be the trigger for the unfolding of a degenerative process. Malignant and degenerative illness is always multifatorial. However, for any degenerative disease to start, there is always a breakdown of the immune responses somewhere in the body.

Real healing comes from within. We all have the potential and capability within us to cope with disease, and a prime object of this book is to explain the background to the likely causes of degenerative diseases, how the body copes and how to bring about the right conditions so that a return to health is often possible. These will include the mental approach as well as ways to feed the body to provide the necessary nutrients, oxygen and vitality and to ensure that what is eaten will actually be of benefit. Most importantly though, Springhill aims to show how one can build up one's immune system, taking into account the person's circumstances (social, financial, political, marital, etc.) – which may have been causal in their developing a diseased state – their lifestyle and in particular their nutrition. The main object of preventive care is to keep the immune system strong.

Cancer, for example, has many causes and there are many influences, both in the internal and external environment, that affect the body and enable the upsurge of conditions to occur in which cancers can flourish. It is interesting to speculate why some people go down with a disease while others, in exactly the same situation, do not. Generally it all comes down to the strength of the person's immune system, which is influenced by heredity, lifestyle, environment, emotions, foods, plus a will to live. This is reflected in lifestyle and can be measured by habits (smoking, drinking, lack of exercise, stressful job, emotional stresses, etc.). Cancer is often, in many ways, a man-made disease. The mere fact of being overweight can often increase the chances of getting cancer, yet it is solely up to the individual to decide whether greed is stronger than the desire to live.

ILLNESS, EMOTIONS AND THE MIND

Illness is thought generally to be something linked with a specific part of the body. Medical specialists have concentrated on breaking down the whole into smaller and smaller parts on which they focus their research, with the result that most treatments are aimed either at suppressing symptoms in that particular area, or cutting out the offending organ or part. It is, however, essential to look at ourselves as whole people, cohabiting with the natural world, and not a collection of parts. People are beginning to realise that one's emotional life influences one's whole being; that fears induce hormonal and nervous changes that affect every cell in the body; and that it may turn out that some emotional and psychological problems will need healing before physical health can be regained.

Psychosomatic illness is one such that originates as a result of, or is aggravated by, an individual's psychological processes. It does not mean that the illness is any less real just because it is not solely physical in origin – if any illness ever is. An ulcer may have originated as a result of, and be aggravated by, anxiety and tension, but this does not make the ulcer any less real. Tissues, organs and functional systems are very susceptible to psychological stress.

The mental attitude of anyone with a serious illness can thus help, or hinder, its progress. The mind affects the physical processes which influence cell behaviour, and this will affect the evolution of a cancer or any other illness. It is therefore important to realise the psychological events which lead to an illness, so that a change in thinking can initiate the first steps towards recovery.

- The patients get a new perspective on their problems; they can act in ways which possibly their upbringing led them to believe were wrong.
- They can learn to show their emotions, for instance assert themselves, and make a conscious decision to alter their behaviour, to become a different kind of person with greater freedom to act.
- The very act of mentally looking forward may actually initiate physical processes that lead towards health.
- The process of recovery leaves the patient mentally and psychologically better than before, and with a different outlook on life.

A positive attitude to treatment being received gives a better idea of how the treatment will turn out than an emphasis on the severity of the disease. It also produces less side effects in the patient.

However, most people are not aware of a link between emotional states and illness. Indeed, Carl Simonton in his book *Getting Well Again* says that some people unconsciously consider there are benefits in illness. Illness often solves problems in people's lives, allowing them to engage in behaviour they would not normally engage in if they were well, e.g. they get increased love and attention, time away from work, reduced responsibility, lessened demands, etc., and it may be the only time when they can experience and accept attention, love and relaxation without feeling guilty.

Illness can, however, also be a trap as it can be used to solve problems; it may appear better to stay ill rather than get better and resume all the responsibilities and worries one had before. It may lead to fantasising about all the care and attention one would receive if one were ill, particularly if it were a terminal illness. This may raise barriers to a person's getting well again and may lead to a point of no return. An illness can be looked on as a temporary protection from daily stresses, and temporary permission to act in more open ways emotionally. This freedom to show feelings as well as emotion needs to be carried on once a person is healthy again in order to prevent a similar situation arising. Illness is an opportunity for the individual to achieve emotional growth; repressed emotions are very damaging and possibly life-threatening.

STRESS AND ILLNESS

Changing behaviour and attitudes may be a matter of life or death and this knowledge can be a powerful motivator for change. Normally a period of stress – with its call-up of protective hormones by the body – is of a comparatively short duration, followed by a period of calm when the body chemistry can relax and get back to normal. Continual stress, which involves the body's alarm system staying on the alert all the time, can produce an excess of adrenaline and other hormones, the metabolic byproducts of which have been found to be major toxins capable of tissue disturbances such as seen in all degenerative diseases. We all suffer stress, perhaps often unknowingly, that affects our immune responses. Recognition of this fact alone can help us enormously, providing action is taken to counter the stresses by removing the causes when identified, or by taking antioxidant agents to counteract the effects of toxins formed as a result of metabolic stress, and by a change in mental attitudes.

There are now clearly recognised links between stress and illness. The emotional response to stress can cause susceptibility to disease. The amount of stress a particular event engenders varies with each individual. Each person has only so much energy to cope with problems – if normal living/working takes up most of one's energy, there is less to spend on keeping oneself well. Emotional stress during the course of any illness may reactivate the disease and even cause the patient to die just when he seemed to be recovering. In contrast, the power of positive emotions can also be harnessed to help the patient regain health; it is possible to learn to control the mental processes which influence a wide variety of physical processes, i.e. 'the mind can relieve illnesses as well as create them'.

In order to sustain good health in a stressful and polluted world, people have to become more aware of the interplay between their bodies, their minds and their emotional/feeling life. In doing so they can learn what they are doing, or are allowing to be done, to their bodies that positively invites disaster. All medication is only a palliative measure to allow nature to work. Gardeners know they can help plants to grow, but they cannot make them grow. Similarly, no amount of medication will heal; it will only palliate. Drugs suppress the symptoms while natural functions take their course and perform the actual task of healing.

SELF-HELP

We all participate in maintaining our own health to some degree (i.e. healing is not only something done to us) through our mental attitudes, our faith in treatment given, our diet, through exercise, in our attitude to smoking, drinking, drugs, etc. Someone with lung cancer who doesn't stop smoking is unlikely to recover, whatever treatment is given; everyone is well aware of the risks involved, and continuing to smoke is tacit acknowledgment that their will to live is very weak. One's attitude of mind, one's will to live, greatly influences the likely benefits from any treatment.

We are all different. Even the foods that are good for one person may not be good for someone else – one man's meat is often another man's poison. Only by understanding the effects of certain foods can one plan an eating pattern that will be right for each individual. Any degenerative illness, if malignant, always shows, through analysis, significant deficiencies of the essential elements for life; in other words there is always malnutrition, not from lack of food but from poor assimilation of nutrients obtained from the food eaten, often as a result of changes in the intestinal flora or degenerative organic and biochemical processes.

These changes are heavily influenced by dietary and environmental factors, and information on what is appropriate in each case is vital in order to aid recovery. What to eat in combination with other foods is also critical, and it may be found that a mere change in the style of eating can accomplish what months or years of drug therapy has been unable to achieve. There may also be actual deficiencies in our diets, notably of elements such as zinc, potassium, magnesium, calcium, which so upset the body's economy that it cannot function efficiently.

In degenerative diseases there are always toxins in the body. Some of these will be acquired from the environment, some from chemicals introduced into our foods through fertilising and spraying crops, from packaging, from other chemicals used in processing foods, from chemicals actually produced in the processing procedure, like the nitro-compounds which are always found in cured meats. These accumulate until they reach the stage when the body cannot metabolise them efficiently and they become toxic or trigger factors in the evolution of disease. Other toxins will be internally created by microorganisms, especially in the gastrointestinal tract. These microorganisms upset the normal working of the intestines to such an extent that partially undigested particles of food get transported into the bloodstream and then toxins travel all over the body, settling in any weak spot. For instance a whiplash accident or other neurological damage in the cervical area could easily be the start of a 'motor' disorder if wandering rogue toxins settle in that area. In cerebral ataxia the cerebellum becomes a mass of fibrous material as a result of the toxins penetrating it, with a lot of granulation developing in the tissues and the coating of the cell walls becoming very fibrous. It is then difficult for oxygen or other nutrients to penetrate the sheath of the cells, which gradually atrophy and die. In arthritis and in muscular dystrophy, as in cerebral ataxia, there is visible hardening of the cells due to damage caused through the influx of too much calcium, as well as peroxidated fats and precipitated salts or sugar particles, seeping in through the cell walls.

With any degenerative illness you have to give yourself a chance to use nutrients. If you give the body nutrients that are hard to break down once ill health is present, you are not helping it at all. You are actually hindering your metabolic processes. Yet a healthy regime does not mean a dull, uninteresting or restricted diet – it only means a different approach to eating and lifestyle.

Prevention is always better than cure. Antioxidants are useful in 'mopping' up oxidising particles but it is more important to turn off the tap rather than to mop up the floor after the damage is done. Cell damage takes place because of the changing character and behaviour of cell components. If there is no fungal, bacterial, or viral over-activity, for example, the oxidation processes are reduced quite significantly. The constant overpopulation of the gut with fungi, bacteria and enteroviruses cause a great deal of fermentative and oxidative processes to take place. Eating the right foods, in the right combination, can correct such metabolic errors.

People who are ill want to go home with a 'package' of instructions and diets; but they must take responsibility themselves and know how to regulate things for themselves in the future. Each person must decide what is best and must know the basis on which to face the future, which may of course include the possibility of dying prematurely. This has to be faced and calmly discussed and appreciated as being just one among many natural and inevitable events in our journey through life.

This ability to take responsibility can only happen through a person knowing how the body works, how foods are used, what foods will help and what will hinder their progress. Everyone has to appreciate how important are mental attitudes, how the mind can affect the physical body, how to relax and meditate and gain peace of mind, how to exercise within the limits of the illness, etc. It may also be useful to get help through spiritual support, hydrotherapy, massage, counselling, Bach flower therapy, homoeopathy. In certain cases osteopathy and chiropractic or acupuncture may help. These are all holistic methods of treating the whole, person, body, mind and spirit. At Springhill the aim is to make available any form of therapeutic care which can at least provide a better quality of life during the last weeks, months or years of someone's life.

SPRINGHILL

The philosophy at Springhill embodies all of these aspects. Patients are encouraged to use their bodies in the best way: to rest when necessary; to undertake creative activities; to relax; to take measures themselves to relieve their pain in non-invasive ways; to understand what is happening in their body so that they can cooperate in any treatment and feel psychologically and mentally prepared for what they are going through.

The underlying belief is that through a change in the way people live, patients come to learn that it is their responsibility and within their power to stay or become healthy. It is essential to live fruitfully, in the present, and not be always living in the past or thinking of the future. For example, about the age of 40 the so-called mid-life crisis often arrives, with an acknowledgment that dreams have not yet materialised. One of the first steps to recovery is the need to identify the attitudes and beliefs that contribute to this feeling of nonachievement and to consider how a person's habitual way of thinking, developed in childhood, may be limiting or impairing the capacity for creative living. Initial goals may have been reached but then comes the feeling 'Is this all?' New challenges need to be made and faced.

Springhill is very much concerned with prevention of disease. Yet, when illness has assailed us, elimination, detoxification and immunity-boosting are the keys to beneficial changes in our health. Hence the emphasis on the integrated healthcare approaches practised and taught at Springhill. The major lesson to be learnt by anyone wanting to take control of their own health is to ensure that toxins are being eliminated; otherwise they have to be stored somewhere, with consequent risk of initiating degenerative processes. Detoxifying the body, the mind and the emotions, may have to be carried out several times. However the aim should be to anticipate breakdowns in the normal functional mechanisms and follow a life that makes it less likely that disease will proliferate. To cut out toxins internally created, while keeping the immune system strong to resist the attacks by external as well as internal factors, is the key. The immune system quickly gets weaker when under siege.

One of the aims of Springhill is to get patients to cut down on foods that are of themselves going to produce a lot of mucus secretions which in turn feed the wrong intestinal microorganisms. The gut then has a chance to release this sticky mucus material, and is given a chance to recolonise with the beneficial flora so that the absorption of food will improve and nutrients will get to the cells throughout the body via the bloodstream and lymphatic fluids.

However, we are all different; it is therefore impossible to stipulate a general diet that everyone should keep to. Guidelines can be given and discussions, sharing experiences, are valuable. To avoid added stress one should never feel alone and struggling; it is better to have an ongoing incentive for change. People do, however, need basic guidelines to start off with. At Springhill the whole process of being ill with a life-threatening illness is handled with the greatest frankness, compassion and friendship. What a blessing is a sense of humour to meet distress with. Laughter is certainly the best medicine – it can literally help increase the production of T cells which are part of our defensive system. So an atmosphere of enthusiasm and gaiety prevails during all gatherings.

Companionship is also vital in the process of healing. Many people find comfort and support in self-help group activities, in sharing, with others similarly placed, their fears, their hopes, their successes and failures in the never-ending search for a better quality of life. They see how others are getting on as a result of taking responsibility for their own health. It is not enough just to meet now and again to share problems and grievances, but to find a basis of sustained friendship where sympathy and understanding represent a vital part of the healing process. Realising what problems other people have makes one often realise how common one's own problems are. Relatives and friends are also tremendously important in the whole healing process, and their education and involvement is as important as that of the patient.

People come to the Springhill Centre with a lot of questions in their minds, two usually being uppermost. Firstly, what is the nature, treatment and prognosis of the illness. This can be answered by specialists within the National Health Service. But the questions most frequently asked by a patient are 'Why do I have to get it?' 'Why me?' How is it that one's normal ability to resist disease has allowed the disease to develop? Much of the help given at the Centre is aimed at putting people in the picture so that they can work out for themselves the answers to these questions. What begins as a journey of transformation for many in a therapeutic setting, such as Springhill, enables each person to find others who are a mirror for their own life's perspectives.

2
ILLNESS CAN BE A BLESSING

To be told by a doctor, when going for some routine tests, that one has a precancerous condition is frightening enough. An actual diagnosis of cancer is shattering. Panic sets in. Why me? What have I done to deserve this? Is this the end? Can it be cured? How long have I got? What will happen to my husband/wife/children without me? And so on.

Relax. The future is in our hands. We must take responsibility for our own health. In some ways this is a fairly simple choice to make, but must be reaffirmed as much as possible to ensure that it becomes a part of our subconscious. And there is also the inbuilt dependence on the medical authorities to overcome. Emile Coue in his wonderful book *Selfmastery Through Conscious Autosuggestion* states that 'it is impossible to think of two things at once' and 'every thought ENTIRELY filling our mind becomes true for us and tends to transform itself into action'. Thus, 'if you can make a sick person think that her trouble is getting better, it will disappear'.

Most people have in their lifestyles – through smoking, drinking, faulty eating habits, stressful business and emotional lives, lack of exercise, etc. – been mainly responsible for their ill-health. Not entirely, of course, as they may have inherited certain weaknesses which have predisposed them towards getting cancer or some other degenerative disease. However, these genetic weaknesses, of themselves, would not have led to their cancer unless they were abusing their body in some way or another, generally quite unconsciously.

Fear is one of the greatest energy-sapping agents, particularly fear of the unknown. Questioning all the time what is going to happen quickly leads to depression. We 'bargain' with our relatives, our friends, our GP, our therapist, saying we are sure they are going to cure us, that we trust them and put our faith in them. We put an almost intolerable burden on them. This is the time when a circle of friendship, support and real companionship is essential. Whether we are healthy or not, we must find time to share with others.

The object of this book is to try and show that the picture is not all black. We can do something about it ourselves. We must all participate in maintaining our own health to some degree and not assume that healing is something done to or for us. We can, first of all, go a long way to preventing the conditions in which cancers flourish. We can reverse any bad habits such as lack of exercise, indulgence in smoking, drinking, drugs, etc. We can eat foods that will provide nourishment for us and not for the unfriendly bacteria which fill our bloodstream with toxins. We can learn to relax and overcome our stresses which are damaging our immune system. And we can develop a positive attitude and expect eventual health, otherwise most treatments will be ineffective.

Coupling this attitude with a knowledge of the body's defence system and knowing ways of coping with stresses can reverse the cancerous cycle. Continued stress results in a feeling of an inability to cope and a feeling of utter hopelessness. Coue, again, says 'we possess within us a force of incalculable power ... and if ... we direct it in a conscious and wise manner, it gives us the mastery of ourselves', and this gives us the necessary self-confidence to take control of our own health.

A prime object of a caring establishment like the Springhill Centre is to give any patient with any form of degenerative disease the opportunity to learn how to boost their immune system physically through appropriate nutrition and changes in lifestyle and, psychologically, with therapeutic activities like painting, sculpture, physiotherapy, massage, specialised counselling, gardening, etc. – in other words through a holistic integrated approach to the care of the whole person. This will include shedding light on things that upset one's metabolism (food and drink toxins, environmental toxins, psychological stresses) and explaining the workings of the body so that one can tackle the problem from the strength of knowledge rather than from one of total ignorance of the defence system of the body. One object of this book therefore is to give a working knowledge of the body and of the mental functions which can play such a great part in recovery. The balance of the immune system must be maintained. If it is upset and the upset is prolonged, then malignancy will set in and cancerous cells will proliferate.

The mental attitude of patients with degenerative diseases is all-important. Surveys have shown that the survival rate after breast cancer operations certainly seems to be affected by the patients' mental attitudes. A 'bad' patient is much more likely to survive than one who accepts his or her fate and leaves everything to the medical team. Optimistic patients who are aggressive towards their disease do far far better than those who merely accept the 'inevitable' as spelt out to them by their friends or their doctor. Furthermore, current research shows how emotions, experiences and attitudes can create physiological change.

Neurological and tissue changes are possible through our attitudes and emotions; an aggressive attitude can actually increase white cell activity and immune system responses. Bernie S. Siegel quotes, in *Love, Medicine and Miracles*, a study which showed that 75 per cent of cancer patients who reacted to their diagnosis with a 'fighting spirit' lived for 10 years or more, compared with 22 per cent who responded with 'stoic acceptance' or feelings of helplessness and hopelessness. He goes on to point out that friends of patients are often told not to give false hope to their ill friends; but there is no such thing as 'false hope'. Hope is a physiological process and can have definite effects on the hormones which activate the immune system.

The healing process starts immediately the patient can see some measure of hope. This, partly, is reflected in how much a person cares about living. I have been appalled, in my practice as a homoeopath, time and time again to come up against people who are ill from smoking-related illnesses and who say to me 'Yes, I know smoking is bad, but I can't give it up.' How can anyone balance a purely addictive habit like smoking against life itself?

A person's level of care for themselves shows up in their efforts, or lack of effort, to stay alive – wearing seat belts, eating the right foods in the right combinations, the natural care and precautions he takes in his daily life, the amount of stress he allows himself to suffer, and the amount of emotion he is willing to show. Again, this is heavily influenced by the people around. The medical staff, friends and relatives can quickly communicate a negative attitude and sense of hopelessness which resolves into a pattern of fear. People who are told they only have a limited time to live will be drained of any real hope of living and such a prophecy will become self-fulfilling.

A serious illness naturally enough focuses our attention on the possibility of dying prematurely. Even in health we should be prepared for and not ignore the fact that we all have to die some time. Death can, however, become just an event in life, just a step into eternity, part of life's journey and not a threatening issue at all. Anyone who can prepare himself to go through the gate of death, through a purification and detoxification process, then knows he is a healthy whole individual. Preparation will involve becoming much more responsible in our actions. It is also necessary to help others to approach death as a journey of transformation, a shedding of the physical body, and to convince them that something lives on.

The value of the warmth of friends and relatives is well illustrated by the work of the comparatively new science of psychoneuroimmunology (PNI), pioneered at Harvard University, and at the Karolinska Institute in Sweden. Scientists there are seeking to find out how to reconstitute the ability of an organism to produce the T cells of the immune system in order to fight invading degenerative or destructive processes. At Harvard, scientists have been able to demonstrate that if an individual is surrounded by warmth – either artificially created by altering environmental conditions, or, above all, by warmth stemming from other individuals such as carers, relatives, friends – the response of that person alters immediately. Within half an hour the level of T-cell production increases measurably and significantly.

This love and warmth from others may represent a very sudden change. The individual concerned may have been starved of warmth and suffered anxieties, fears, deep-seated problems and perhaps loneliness. All of this would have altered the normal bodily processes and impaired the functional responses of the glands, which would have in turn been secreting toxic substances, leading to the production of free-radical toxins as byproducts of glandular metabolism (see Chapter 19). This phenomenon is something that we must acknowledge in order to see where, in our own lives, warmth can be generated to help others and to help ourselves. In the scientific trials that lead to this conclusion, support from families, counsellors, psychologists and other carers was used. Other means of generating a total atmosphere of warmth included artistic activities, music, touch, aromatherapy, etc., all of which served to help accelerate the production of T cells as part of the improved immune responses of the individual.

There are however some positive benefits to be got from a serious illness. In fact illness can be a blessing. It often gives one enormous opportunities to reconsider one's lifestyle, to reconcile oneself to the future, to undergo change and to help those who are nearest to undergo change too. It gives us an opportunity to find out about ourselves in a totally new context. It gives us time to look at the quality of our life, time to be creative, time to consider whether there is enough time to relax and do the things one really wants to do, rather than those things that are expected of us. What, in fact, do we want to do? It gives us time to plough through the maze of information that is constantly bombarding us, to find something that is going to suit us as individuals, so that it will alter significantly the pattern we set for ourselves.

For the last 50 years health care has been delivered to us. Once we are ill, there are the health services to serve us whenever needed. We may go on for years with headaches, the odd pains, discomfort, or just general malaise, and we think that it is normal to have minor complaints. Then, the day comes when we feel that these little symptoms have been going on long enough. We go to see our local doctor and, suddenly, we are faced with the trauma of illness, which often shakes us to the core. Perhaps surgery is offered. After what is often a disabling illness, we come up against enormous complexities which force us to alter dramatically the patterns of 'normal' living. First of all we have to become conversant with the illness and know what to look for as the illness progresses; as we start to recover we need to know if there is going to be any sort of life afterwards. What kind of a life will it be?

At centres like Springhill there must be opportunities for exploring these questions, listening to others who are in, or have been in, the same sort of situation, and above all to find time and space for ourselves in our busy lives to explore how better to help ourselves; time to become more conversant with our own bodies and how they work, how our mental responses affect our physical body, how to cope with our families during the initial trauma. In fact, how to live now. How to relax. How to 'cope'.

We need to consider what mental problems may be lying behind our physical ailments, which are distorting our responses. We need to see whether we can make any contribution to the life of someone else who is dominated by their illness, particularly someone who has just been diagnosed as having a degenerative and possibly life-threatening disease. They will almost certainly be going through the trauma of shock, bitterness, anger, bewilderment and disbelief that comes when first hearing the diagnosis.

A time of enforced inaction, with little prospect of ever regaining full health, gives us a further golden opportunity – a chance, and an incentive, to think about healing. Everyone has the potential, and the ability, to heal. The body is composed of different forms of energy, activated in many different ways. This energy flows through all living systems and is always in a state of movement. If it is blocked or interrupted in any way it causes an imbalance, and clearance of these blockages is the basis of techniques such as acupuncture. The flow of energy is said to be regulated by the seven chakras or centres in the body, each of which is associated with specific parts of the body. Each has specific functions and each is connected with the functioning of specific glands and nerve groups. When these chakras are 'balanced', then healing takes place. But this can only happen when one has a positive mental outlook, which is something that is under our conscious control. It only remains for us to be single-minded in our pursuit of total health and to give up all thoughts of disease, all activities that provide more than minimal stress, and be aware that the change in outlook will require changes in habitual patterns of behaviour.

Illness often gives one the time to consider the future. It is a 'journey of transformation' between what we are and what we would like to become, when we use the unawakened potential that lies deep within us. It gives us the time to create the precipitating factors to bring about the advent of those things that have been longed for; to contemplate and produce creative thoughts about what we long for and how to get it.

Even when fully healthy one should not feel guilty about making time and space to do the creative things that one would find fulfilling. It is essential, as it makes one a more balanced and enriched individual. However, there is really no necessity to get ill in order to have the time to think about this. It may be argued that perhaps a person will set his goals too high, but God moves in a mysterious way and, providing one is watching out for opportunities, they will appear in ways that perhaps would not be recognised as such if one were not consciously on the lookout. And this will only happen after a period of concentrated thought. One often needs an illness to bring us back to human values.

3
WHAT IS CANCER?

Let us start with some definitions:

- Cancer is a whole body disease, showing up as an abnormal cellular proliferation, a new growth, called a neoplasm or tumour, which is continually growing at the expense of normal cells.
- A tumour is an abnormal lump of tissue. Its growth is uncoordinated with normal tissue and continues to grow after the initial stimulus of growth is over. Tumours 'contain' or confine cancer cells. But excising tumours, or radiation therapy, can lead to metastases.
- A metastasis is a secondary cancer formed from cells which have detached themselves from the primary growth and grouped themselves together in another location where the conditions are suitable, e.g. where a vein or artery has been blocked.

A tumour is hard and does not yield to, or pit on, pressure and is generally localised in one spot. A cyst (or oedema) on the other hand is filled with fluid and yields to, and pits, on pressure, and may cover a large area. Inflammations have redness, pain and heat: tumours do not.

BENIGN TUMOURS

Benign tumours do not grow much and remain localised, i.e. do not appear in other parts of the body (metastasise). They do not normally recur after excision and they do not normally produce haemorrhages or ulcerations.

Benign tumours are normally distinguished by the letters -oma being added to the name of the tissue concerned, e.g. fibroma is a tumour of fibrous tissue. Some exceptions are:

- A sarcoma is a malignant tumour forming in connective tissues, muscle, bone and cartilage.
- A carcinoma, the most common malignant cancer, is a tumour of the epithelial cells that cover tissues and line body cavities, the stomach, the lungs, the gastrointestinal tract and which also occur in glandular organs such as the breast.

MALIGNANT TUMOURS

Malignant tumours have a rapid growth and infiltrate neighbouring tissues.

- They absorb nourishment of the host.
- They produce toxic products.
- They may form open ulcers, and haemorrhages are very common.
- They have the ability to spread to other parts of the body (metastasise).
- They tend to recur after excision.
- They are characterised by growth extending along lines of least resistance, destroying normal tissue. The word cancer (or the crab) is given because of the crablike extensions of the cells into the surrounding tissues, thus making it difficult to hold in the malignant cells.
- The malignant cells are motile (able to move round the body) through reduced adhesiveness, due to deficiencies of certain essential electrolytes in the cell membranes: cells of benign tumours are firmly anchored to one another.

Malignant cancer cells can invade blood vessels (veins more than arteries), and therefore those organs subject to main venous drainage become sites of cancer, e.g. lungs, liver, axial bones (sarcomas are commonly spread in this way). The spread in kidneys, endocrine glands and bone marrow is due to arterial embolisms or blockages caused by undissolved material getting stuck in a vein or artery; this material is invaded by tumour cells, and the whole thing then detaches and forms tumour emboli which get carried round the arteries. Malignant cells may spread through serous cavities, e.g. from stomach to ovaries, they may spread as a result of an operation, and they can spread through natural passages, e.g. malignant cells may be carried along bowels, bronchus, vagina and ureter, where they can implant on the epitheleal surface and form a new growth.

Malignant tumours often cause progressive weakness, malnutrition, emaciation and general debility called cachexia.

LEUKAEMIAS AND LYMPHOMAS

Leukaemia is an uncontrolled overproduction of white blood cells which lowers plasma nutrient levels. It is thus a cancer of the blood. It is a chronic disease in which the blood's white corpuscles are considerably increased. Anaemia often accompanies this disease. There is also likely to be an enlargement of the spleen and probably of the lymph glands all over the body.

Malaria and syphilis are said to be possible causes of leukaemia. Syphilis is one of Samuel Hahnemann's (the founder of homoeopathy) 'miasms' or hereditary tendencies to certain diseases and if this is the cause it narrows down the choice of homoeopathic remedies to use. The anaemia and general inflammation of the lymphatic glands also suggest a background of gonorrhoea (the sycotic miasm in homoeopathic terms) for which there is another range of homoeopathic remedies.

Cytomegalo virus has also been implicated as a cause, and there is now evidence that changes in the body's electromagnetism, possibly as a result of living or working near high-voltage power lines, can also be a cause of leukaemia, particularly in children. Continuous exposure to low-ionising radiations is now acknowledged to be implicated in the evolution of neoplasias and genetic mutations.

Symptoms of leukaemia will include gradual swelling of the abdomen, shortness of breath, painless enlargement of the spleen, the glands in the neck, armpits, etc., plus a pallor if anaemic. There may be dropsy (oedema, or excess fluid in the tissues) of the legs, some fever, perhaps diarrhoea alternating with constipation. There are often short remissions when the glands and spleen appear normal, but after a relapse the condition is worse than before.

Children with leukaemia always show signs of candidiasis and therefore often require anti-candida diet and treatment. Otherwise routinely conventional treatment can cure up to 50 per cent of childhood leukaemias.

In leukaemias the most important area of trouble is the portal vein, which collects veinous blood from the gastrointestinal tract and organs to evacuate toxins. As the toxins are in the blood which goes all over the body, leukaemia is therefore a systemic disease and is not contained in a small 'package' such as a tumour. Post mortems confirm that in leukaemics the portal vein is always infiltrated by fungi, streptococci, other bacteroids and viral organisms.

Vitamin C has been found to be lacking in leukaemics as it becomes locked up in the excessive numbers of white cells. Up to 25 grams a day can be taken to redress the balance. Note that easy bruising means a person is probably short of vitamin C.

Two similar forms of cancer are lymphomas and multiple myelomas. Lymphomas are tumours in lymph tissue, often in overweight people who eat a lot of dairy products. Multiple myelomas are rare bone marrow tumours.

GENERAL COMMENTS

Hippocrates, some 2,000 years ago, said that cancer was a general body disease which eventually caused a local outbreak in the form of a growth. It is therefore a constitutional disease and cures should come only through constitutional remedies and treatment aimed at the whole body and personality.

Cancer cannot be caught; it is completely uninfectious. However it can be spread around the body, most commonly via the lymphatic or blood channels, which can carry it anywhere in the body. The pattern of spread will depend on normal drainage routes of the lymph, e.g. carcinoma of the breast will metastasise first to internal mammary nodes and then to axillary nodes in the armpit.

Tumours and cysts often form when a woman is pregnant because too much residual metabolic material, for example gluten and fat (i.e. very long-chain saturated fatty acids), is in the milk which is not flowing properly through the mammary gland conduits. This will very likely give rise to fungal, bacterial and viral infestation as well.

But our focus of concern should not be with processes of one part of the body only, but with the whole body – the blood, the lymph which drains the toxins out of the blood, the bone structure, even the posture of the body and how we carry ourselves is important. We are to be concerned with ourselves as whole human beings and not just as a collection of parts.

Illness has so much to do with our attitudes and emotions and how we react to life and the conditions of which we are constantly victims, right back to our forebears and the types of culture in which we have been brought up. It is a search, a quest, to try and understand the evolution of the disease by studying the various facets leading up to its emergence. It is however important, whenever we are ill, to understand a little of the mechanics of the ailment.

4
THE CAUSES OF CANCER

There are a number of trigger factors that result in a person getting cancer, and many of them relate to:

- Faulty nutrition – apart from a grossly imbalanced diet, this may imply an excess of drugs, or an intake of nitrates, chemical fertilisers and sprays which are present in the food we eat. It does not necessarily mean a faulty diet, though, but rather a lack of nutrients available to the cells or a supply of the wrong nutrients.
- Environmental pollution – environmental triggers will include carcinogens (chemicals that cause cancer) such as coal tar, hydrocarbons in cigarettes and carbon tetrachloride used for cleaning.
- Emotional and behavioural stressors.

VARIOUS CAUSES

- The diet, of course, may be very poor allowing the body to be filled with excess fat, sugars, undigested or only partly digested proteins, resulting in constipation or diarrhoea, which often leads to auto-intoxication or self-poisoning.
- There may be some obvious gaps in the diet which result in a deficiency of potassium. This may be caused by the consumption of an excess of salt (sodium). There is a very delicate sodium/potassium balance in the body which, if disturbed, will lead to trouble. There is potassium inside the body cells, while sodium is outside the cells, in the body fluids. Potassium is an oxygen attractant and oxygen is absolutely essential in all cells. If there is an excess of sodium, some will infiltrate the cells and will cancel out the effect of the potassium.
- Stresses and worry use up potassium phosphate in the blood, cells, nerves and brain, so stress can, quite directly, produce a potassium shortage.
- Genetics play their part, too, as genetically altered cells may have been inherited and their weaknesses will show up, particularly with advancing age.

- Radiation of various kinds may trigger off the evolution of cancerous cells. The radiation may be from X-rays, television sets, VDUs, faulty microwave ovens, radioactive paint (as in watches with luminous dials, which can produce bone sarcomas), fallout from nuclear disasters, ionising radiations from overhead power lines, etc.

- Dysbiosis (an alteration in the flora of the intestines), which particularly includes fungal and bacterial overgrowth, can produce very powerful carcinogens. Fermentation as a result of an unbalanced diet, or a diet of foods that feed the microorganisms rather than the person, will produce a breakdown of oxygen bonds which will quickly lead to factors which cause malignant disease.

- Surgery, even a simple biopsy, can introduce carcinogens (mould toxins) into the bloodstream and contaminate the entire system, producing an outbreak of infection in one or another weakened spot. After surgery of malignant tumours the immune system is very weak, so extra care is then necessary to avoid systemic contamination by mould.

- Chronic physical irritation of a certain part of the anatomy can produce cancers, e.g. cancer of the lips of pipe smokers, cancer of gums due to ill-fitting dentures, cancer of the cervix due to abrasive sexual intercourse and too frequent pregnancies, cancer of the skin due to excessive suntanning.

- Shortages of minerals and vitamins may so weaken the body that it falls prey to any toxins. And shortage of vitamin C, in particular, as it protects the body from the toxin acetaldehyde in cigarette smoke, which is a trigger for heart disease and lung cancer.

- Pancreatic enzyme deficiencies have been considered one of the most significant causes of cancer (see below).

Nearly all of the above add up to a weakening of the immune system. Anyone with a strong functioning immune system is unlikely to get a degenerative disease, as the natural bodily defences will then be able to cope with invaders.

The place and house one lives in can have a very deleterious effect on one's health. There is now sufficient evidence to suggest there are cancer localities where radiations from the earth cause an increased incidence of cancer. These areas are named geopathic zones and are found over geological faults, underground streams and other moving subterranean water such as sewers, mines, etc. It has been shown that there is a change in the earth's magnetic field strength in these geopathic zones, with an increased level of electromagnetic radiation in the microwave range and an increase in gamma radiation, all of which can upset the delicate electromagnetism of the body's nerve fibres, etc. There are instances of houses in which a number of people have had cancer over the years (e.g. radon gases in granite houses) – too large a number to have happened coincidentally.

There may be a chronic shortage of a certain mineral in the local area from which vegetables and fruits are bought, and this can upset the natural balance in the body. Or the local water supply may be highly contaminated with aluminium, lead, chlorine, fluoride, algae, or nitrates, or the house one lives in may be full of damp and mould which encourages microbial growth.

American research has shown that about 75 per cent of people who get cancer have certain characteristics in common (often low self-esteem, a sense of rejection, inability to form stable personal relationships, self-pity), all of which could possibly be traced to an emotional instability when a child, to a period of loneliness and lack of satisfactory family relationships. Recent bereavements are also thought to bring about the conditions which can trigger off cancers.

So, there is no single cause for cancer – which comes in various forms anyway. The main line of defence is to keep fit mentally as well as physically, to eat the right foods, in the right combinations, and to avoid unnecessary stresses or learn how to deal with them calmly, whether physical, mental or emotional, and to recognise other stresses as being such.

FAULTY NUTRITION

Faulty nutrition, particularly an excess of protein and fatty acids, is thought to be at the root of all cancers, according to all the leading doctors who advocate a natural way of curing and preventing cancer. Rudolf Breuss, for example, contends that cancers cannot live without some protein and, by starving them of protein, many can be destroyed in about 40 days (see Chapter 25). There are, however, differences of opinion as to what foods specifically are harmful or beneficial. For example, breast cancer is said to be directly related to the amount of animal fat and proteins eaten, bowel cancer is often related to the amount of red meat and proteins eaten, while lung cancer is related to tobacco smoke and bovine dairy products. Bowel and breast cancer can also be associated with selenium deficiency.

Calories measure the amount of energy stored in food, mainly in the carbohydrates. (Carbohydrates are often abbreviated as CHO, because they consist of carbon, hydrogen and oxygen.) Empty calories is the term for those foods that supply energy (calories) but none of the other nutrients necessary for their use by the body; therefore vitamins, minerals and other nutrients have to be 'stolen' in order to use up these empty calorie foods. Typical empty-calorie foods are white sugar, white flour, processed fats and starches, potatoes without their skins, in contrast to unrefined carbohydrates – whole grains, brown rice, peas, beans, lentils, nuts, dried fruits, fresh fruits and vegetables – which contain a balanced range of nutrients. In addition, the less refined the food, the more slowly is it used by the body; this therefore does not require an abnormally high level of the hormone insulin in order to bring down an exaggerated level of blood sugar.

Any food taken in excess of the energy requirements, e.g. excessive protein consumption, will be turned into oxidated waste matter which creates surplus tissue stores of fat, fluids, hormones etc. (causing cellulite bulges). But to do this, the body needs extra nutrients, which it may well be short of, in order to store these extra calories. The result is that one gets a feeling of being unwell.

A body needs three things, and any treatment must take into account all three:

- A sufficient intake of healthy foods, vitamins, minerals, amino acids and enzymes.
- Necessary proper usage by the body of these nutrients; this will involve the proper combinations of foods that act synergistically with each other.
- All waste materials must be efficiently eliminated or else the body will slowly poison itself; in other words the body will suffer with auto-intoxication.

IMBALANCE BETWEEN POTASSIUM, SODIUM AND CALCIUM

Cancer patients are always short of bio-available potassium, although this shortage may be a cause or a result of the chemical changes in the body. A shortage of available potassium can show up as:

- Mental depression – this shows up first.
- Catarrh or sinusitis.
- Painful trapezius muscles (up the side of the neck; i.e. 'stiff neck').
- Cold hands and feet through lack of circulation. Note that toxic blood or lymph fluid makes the thyroid react; this governs the activity of the liver, kidneys and spleen, so all these organs can be

affected and illnesses in them may be part of the arthritic, or cancerous, picture.

- Premature grey hair.

Foods rich in potassium are bananas, avocados, celery, apples, potatoes in their jackets, coconuts, dandelions, watercress and spinach. Supplementation may be by use of potassium chloride (as in salt substitutes).

A major function of the adrenal glands is to maintain the body's sodium/potassium balance. If however a person has hypoadrenia (poorly performing adrenals), the body may retain an excess of potassium. Symptoms of hypoadrenia are:

- Extreme fatigue in the mornings, improving as the day wears on.
- Blood pressure which does not rise on standing up.
- Hypoglycaemia – low blood sugar level.
- Asthma, allergies.
- All those symptoms get worse when drinking coffee.

On the other hand, hyperactivity of the adrenals will produce excess cortisone which holds up the excretion of sodium, which then builds up and becomes toxic. With cancer, potassium is leached and sodium invades the cells.

Nutritional changes to be considered are as follows.

- Use naturally available salts.
- Consume a low-fat diet.
- Drastically reduce the consumption of sugar.

A detoxification process is essential once the potassium and oxidising ions and enzymes get into the cancer cells, killing them by taking away the condition of fermentation under which they exist. There will then be a mass of dead cell material to be excreted.

EXCESS OF SALT

This is a natural corollary of an imbalance with potassium.

Dr Maud Fere, in her book *Does Diet Cure Cancer?*, suggests that cancer may be linked with the response of the body to too much sodium which comes from the diet and also from fertilisers like sodium nitrate used on green vegetables.

Sodium chloride, in contact with water, breaks down in the body to hydrochloric acid and sodium hydroxide (i.e. caustic soda, which is an alkali). The hydrochloric acid is removed from the blood and used in the digestion process. The sodium hydroxide that is left combines with carbonic acid (CO_2) in the blood, forming sodium carbonate, which will mainly be reformed into sodium hydroxide. There is therefore a certain amount of sodium hydroxide left in the blood whenever excess salt is eaten.

Sodium hydroxide (caustic soda) is an irritant to the cells it comes in contact with and the body neutralises it with lactic acid, produced by an anaerobic fermentation process (metabolism in the absence, or limited supplies, of oxygen) which is very common in 'embryonic' cells – fast growing cells capable of producing large quantities of lactic acid. These embryonic cells are similar, if not identical, to cancer cells. Therefore reducing the amount of salt intake is likely to reduce the number of embryonic cells produced and, by implication, the number of potentially altered or malignant cell changes.

Bihari, in his book *Homoeopathic Insight Into Cancer — Causes, Treatment and Cure*, says 'In cancer cases, invariably, without exception, there is sodium toxicity which ... replaces calcium and makes it deficient, leading to cardiac trouble' and 'when potassium also becomes deficient, there is calcification at localised spots in the form of benign tumours or neoplasm'. Bihari suggests that homoeopathic adrenalin 200 fortnightly can help to eliminate sodium from the system.

To test if there is excessive sodium in the blood, take red litmus paper and place it under the upper lip next to the gum. Leave it for a few minutes and if it turns blue, then there is too much alkali in the body. Normally it should only turn very slightly blue. High alkalinity of the blood, shown by abnormal blueness of the litmus paper when tested, may be a sign of a precancerous state.

Sodium hydroxide irritation may cause a burning sensation in one or more places of the body, although the affected part will feel cold to the touch. This also is a sign of the possibility that cancer may follow; for example, skin cancer may be caused through sunburn, which releases caustic soda at the site of the burn. However, if fluorides (sodium fluoride) accumulate in the body they cannot be removed; so cancer, if caused by excess sodium through fluorides, cannot be reversed – surely a compelling reason to cut out salt from the diet.

PANCREATIC ENZYME DEFICIENCIES

Enzymes are proteins which control the biochemical reactions in the body, every metabolic function requiring a different enzyme. Within the gastrointestinal tract, the gut, a variety of enzymes are secreted into the food mass; their task is to break down the large food molecules – the sugars, carbohydrates, fats and proteins – into smaller and smaller molecules until they are eventually small enough to pass across the gut wall and into the bloodstream. They can then be distributed around the body and incorporated into the body's processes.

One of the principal sources of these digestive enzymes is the pancreas, but it is thought that these pancreatic enzymes have a dual task, not only of digesting proteins in the food we eat, but also of trying to digest 'foreign' unwanted cells such as in tumours. These enzymes can also be supplemented through enzyme preparations that can be taken by mouth to boost the body's supply, enzymes such as:

- Bromelain – this is anti-inflammatory and is useful in post-operative healing.
- Antioxidant enzymes like superoxide dismutase (SOD), glutathione peroxidase, methionine reductase and catalase.

Such enzymes can now be enteric coated to ensure they pass through the acidity of the stomach without being degraded, allowing them to act where they are needed in the small intestine.

Cancer cells, initially freely circulating in the blood, are attacked by these enzymes which destroy their protective mucus coating, making it possible for the normal immune defences to work – providing, of course, there are enough pancreatic enzymes. Dr Kelley has stated that a 'malignancy indicates an active pancreatic enzyme deficiency'. And the most significant cause of pancreatic enzyme deficiency is excessive undigested protein.

Cancer does not happen suddenly and would probably not happen at all if sufficient pancreatic enzymes were present, to break down protein.

Cancers that start as a result of a deficiency of pancreatic enzymes mostly due to microbial infestation of vital organs have some peculiar characteristics unlike other cancers, e.g. a lot of excessive gas, unusual mental states, depression and a change from being normally happy and cheerful to being depressed, etc.

The pancreas cannot manufacture enough enzymes to digest a heavy intake of foods like milk, cheese, meat, fish, eggs, etc. (all of which are often denatured by heat treatment), and have enough enzymes left over to digest cancer cells or other foreign proteins. The body must however have some protein because if it does not get sufficient protein it will rob the muscle system, which will result in muscle weakness, extreme loss of energy, skin hanging in loose folds (which may become permanent). Indeed pancreatic enzymes are protein, and therefore the body must be fed adequate protein for the pancreas to produce its protein. It is important, therefore, to have a low protein intake rather than no protein, especially easily digested proteins.

The same enzymes used in the digestion of meat are used in the digestion of cancer cells, so eating less meat means more enzymes are free to digest malignant cells. Meat of large mammals also has disproportionately large amounts of sex hormones which become initiators and precursors of malignant cell changes. Raw organic lambs' liver (a good blood builder) may be used by all cancer patients if taken before noon each day. Most protein should be taken by lunchtime – this gives about six hours for the digestive enzymes to work, which then have the remaining 18 hours in which to concentrate on digesting waste matter. The liver can be put in the blender with carrots, or tomato juice as a morning 'pep up' drink. It is especially good for leukaemia and lymphomas.

Milk is too high in protein and its digestion requires too many pancreatic enzymes, so not more than 8 oz per day of milk or milk products should be taken. It is advisable to have it in the form of yoghourt made with sheep or goat's milk, as the bacteria in yoghourt predigest milk protein; if this causes too much mucus, take 1 ounce of liquid acidophilus (the bacteria that makes yoghourt) to maintain friendly bacterial flora in the gut.

Any sugar (or any sugar products) similarly gives the pancreas too much work when it should be digesting toxins and cancers.

OXYGEN DEFICIENCY IN THE CELLS

Otto Warburg discovered that cancer cells are able to obtain their energy without the use of oxygen. Normal cells obtain most of their energy from the use of oxygen, but if there is no oxygen the cells convert to malignant cells very quickly.

Dr Robert Olney considers that 'blocked oxidation' is the prime cause of malignant, viral, bacterial and allergic diseases. The oxidation process (respiration) of living cells is essential for health, but blockage can come about through injury, various toxic substances and lack of oxygen. A lack of oxygen (anaerobic conditions) leads to fermentation of the sugars of the cells in order to produce the required energy. Viruses, and organisms such as *Candida albicans* (a yeast), grow profusely under these conditions.

Dr Olney treated such cases with intravenous injections of the patient's own blood which had been irradiated by ultraviolet light; this rapidly increases the oxygen absorption of the patient, bringing the blood oxygen up to normal levels. Dr C. Moerman increased oxygenation through increased circulation by prescribing citric acid, 15–20 grams dissolved in 250 ml of water – a desertspoonful of this three times a day. Citric acid helps blood circulation by combating oedema, fermentation and alkali in the blood. Dr Moerman also recommends dry red wine (300 g) plus a 3 per cent solution of iodine, which he found increased oxygenation by dilating fine blood vessels; it combines with albumen to give it the function of thyroxin which controls the rate of oxidation.

Dr Issels pointed out that the diet of cancer patients must contain very little fermentable carbohydrates, e.g. sugar or starch, which breaks down to glucose, since cancer cells need to ferment sugar to get their energy. Diet should also include items which encourage aerobic conditions, e.g. fresh green juices and fresh lambs' liver juice. Shortage of the B vitamins and magnesium will slow down the aerobic oxidation process. Magnesium is a catalyst which is required in the breakdown of glucose into CO_2, water and energy. (Note that fluorides inactivate magnesium and encourage anaerobic respiration and eventually leading up to the production of cancer cells.)

Lactic acid is used to neutralise sodium hydroxide formed by the breakdown of sodium chloride. It is produced under anaerobic conditions from the breakdown of glucose WITHOUT magnesium. If not required, the lactic acid is then returned to the liver and reconverted, with the use of much energy, back to glucose, which cancer cells in turn convert to lactose, again using energy. The result is that the body gets tired through the continual use of energy in non-productive measures.

Toxic poisons in the body accumulate in various spots and use up body oxygen, so the higher the concentration of these poisons, the more chance there is of a cancerous process developing. Cancer is the result of long-standing toxicity of the body.

Damage to cells, perhaps by surgery, traumatic injury, burns or biopsy, will encourage the formation of embryonic cells to repair the damage. Unfortunately these cells operate without oxygen, and therefore encourage fermentation and the growth of defective cells.

Increasing aerobic respiration slows down cancer growth. Copper and other heavy metals are not wanted by cancer cells, so if copper can be introduced into them, aerobic respiration increases.

HEREDITARY INFLUENCES

If you are born with a specific genetic handicap you are going to inherit systemic weaknesses, such as a weakness in the gut. This will be accentuated if both parents have the same weakness (such as a weak thyroid or a weakness in the intestinal lining).

For example, if both parents have a weak duodenal or ileal

membrane (both are areas of the small intestine) there are several possibilities. If there is a weak lining to the gut which allows toxins to migrate to the head area of the foetus, then the next generation is likely to be affected by psychological illness (research carried out by the University of Bangor, funded by the Schizophrenia Foundation). If just one of the parents (especially the mother) has a weak gut lining allowing transportation of toxins, the weakness goes to the digestive tract, possibly resulting in coeliac disease. Genetic prints are now very much under scrutiny to help identify patterns of disease.

DECAY OF THE GUT-BLOOD BARRIER

One of the major problems of modern times is that in most of us the small intestine gets so permeable and infected by the wrong micro-organisms that it allows the transportation of all kinds of toxins into the blood. The blood sends them on into the lymph, which in turn sends them to the skin, the kidneys, the lung, etc., and all the organs of elimination have to carry a heavy extra load because the gut is not functioning properly or carefully discriminating between what is true food and what isn't. The kind of illness we are going to develop (apart from ailments arising out of accidents of one kind or another) depends on where the genetic weaknesses are and where the toxicity builds up.

STRESS

Emotional stress is probably the most insidious, as well as being the most hidden, cause of disease. It can be useful to identify some personal crisis between 6 and 18 months prior to the disease being diagnosed; this could very well have been the trigger that set in motion a weakening of the immune system. Was this crisis one that was thrust on the individual? Was it a result of being locked in such a situation? If so it may be necessary to identify beliefs or behaviour patterns which may need changing; otherwise there may be a recurrence of the cancer (assuming there has been a remission or possible cure). Perhaps there may have been the loss of a close family member. The way we react to stress is more important than the stress itself.

Cancer is often a reaction to a set of circumstances that have so weakened the body's immune defence system that it cannot cope with what would otherwise be an easily overcome invasion of toxins. We all live under stress of one kind or another and this stress can take many forms. One step to be taken in our recovery programme is to recognise the stresses and to tackle them positively. Illness can be a time of opportunity, a time to review one's life and its stresses, and recognise the damage that unmanaged stress may be doing to us. Appreciating how we are, perhaps unconsciously, trying to cope with them is a vital start towards overcoming them.

The most traumatic events in one's life often have far-reaching consequences and it is well established that the death of a spouse is often the trigger for the appearance of a cancer some 18 months to two years later. Other disturbing experiences like divorce, loss of a job, shattering of a life-long ambition, etc., all take their toll on the immune system and may weaken it so much that the body is unable to resist invasive toxins. So grief, fears, worries – emotional or financial – have to be consciously acknowledged and examined as if from the outside. One can always see that other people's worries are not really justified or are not as bad as they would like you to think they are; perhaps our worries and fears look the same to someone else and are therefore not worth getting into a state over. Artists can always see what is wrong with other people's pictures but cannot see what is glaringly wrong in the perspective in their own pictures.

A calm acceptance of a stress factor will help to put it into its right perspective. Bottling up a stressful worry, grief or fear starts off a chain of physical and chemical reactions. The body reacts to trauma with its 'fight or flight' mechanism, producing adrenaline and converting carbohydrates stored in the muscles and liver to provide the necessary energy to fight, or flee. Unfortunately if the threatened danger does not materialise and our responsive energy is not used, but is repressed, then bodily symptoms of disease start to appear, perhaps as a stiff neck, difficulty in breathing, permanent sinusitis, digestive problems, lower back ache, pain in the shoulders, insomnia, anxiety for no reason at all, or almost any other ailment. These are all merely the body's way of telling us that something is wrong; these symptoms should not be repressed by drugs but the cause should be brought out and treated.

Resentment is one of the most destructive emotions one can carry around. When we artificially keep alive the original feeling of anger, etc., we keep on resurrecting the actual physical responses. Lymphocyte production (the first line of defence of the immune system) is then reduced as a result of stress, thus weakening the defence capability of the body.

Unattended stress goes on as if nothing has happened. If perhaps someone flies off the handle at the least provocation, he is generating a high level of carcinogenic material in the body because of the byproducts of glandular metabolism – particularly the adrenal secretions which are produced as a result of any acute stress response. Adrenaline byproducts have pointed crystalline forms which can perforate the membranes of cells, which then begin to oxidate (the oxides begin to be formed in the cell). At the point of wounding the cell starts to leak little bits of plasma; this is called cell blebbing (it might be more accurate to call it cell bleeding, as what is coming out of the cell is plasma), and it does this to protect and heal itself. In such a situation, where an external agent has come and caused havoc with a living system, or where there is damage in a small cluster of cells but no repair material is coming in, perhaps because of a poor diet, then you have a potentially cancerous milieu.

Management of stress is thus essential for anyone who has a malignancy; even when they have a benign tumour it is important to control stress because if the level of toxins grows, then those benign tumours can become malignant. However, the actual presence of cancerous cells does not necessarily mean that cancer will develop, only that when the immune system is weakened in any way, then they will be more likely to proliferate.

A feeling of hopelessness and helplessness is extremely debilitating and produces those physical changes in the body that make it probable that normal cell production will break down and cancerous cells may proliferate. It is possible – in fact it is essential – to change one's mental attitude to stresses because it is only in this way that beneficial physical changes can be activated.

The amount of stress that a particular event engenders varies with each individual. To cope with stress requires a lot of energy and there may not be enough left over for everyday living – or vice versa, in which case the stress cannot be met and overcome. Hans Selye, in his book *The Stress of Life*, defines stress as 'the nonspecific response of the body to any demand'. It has a general effect on the whole body, perhaps giving a feeling of just being tired all the time for no apparent reason. The response is general but the end effect is for the weakest part of the body to succumb.

We can help ourselves in many ways. Environmental allergens constitute 70 per cent of triggers, whose effects will be aggravated if we are suffering from stress. For instance, one easy way of helping oneself is to hoover mattresses, curtains and chairs to get rid of house dust mites. Use biodegradable washing powders. Replace aluminium pans with stainless steel or copper pans. Install an efficient water filtering device, preferably one that works on the reverse osmosis principle which takes out the majority of potentially dangerous substances.

Environmental triggers include chemicals such as those in air fresheners, cleaning agents, car fumes, weedkillers, agrochemicals, tobacco, effluents; and work and household appliances like tubular lighting, television sets and photocopiers. Many activities have vibrations that produce toxic responses in a person if they are sensitive to noise – the vibrations go right through them, and they secrete steroids and chemical toxins. Other influences are airborne microorganisms such as fungi, toxins that are byproducts of plant and animal metabolism, chemicals in plastic containers, interiors of cars, furnishings. Today's environment has become highly toxic; this insidious danger we often do not notice or appreciate.

Cooking often destroys vitamins, enzymes, amino acids and all principal nutrients, and also impairs the binding of the minerals. Normally minerals and metals present in food are attached to enzymes and other proteins and are biologically active, but as soon as you cook or heat-treat or irradiate foodstuffs, minerals and metals, they become biologically inert and chemically active, and may attach themselves very easily to other harmful chemical bonds. A combination of such chemicals, some of which may be bad, with a heavier molecular weight, is then formed.

Much stress is anticipatory worry. We are often afraid of what might happen and it is useful to consider some of the alternative ways of overcoming such worries. Firstly one needs to consider whether there is any rational reason why such an event should happen. It is necessary to look at the problem as if it were one brought up by a friend asking for your advice. The onlooker sees more of the game and, in the case of worries, can see more clearly whether there is any substance in them. Think of what the worst possible result could be. Are the facts of the situation really likely to produce such dire results? Have you perhaps been in similar situations in the past and been able to cope? Why then should you not cope with the new problems?

Unless stresses of a non-physical kind are removed, or the body learns how to cope with them, little can be done nutritionally. There is still a constrictive unconscious process going on. Stress equals constriction equals seizing up, under stress, in a metabolic functional sense. Stress interrupts all the metabolic processes to a point.

There are two types of stresses – internal, from our own metabolism, and external. However, from the point of view of the cell itself, all toxins are external, unless we have a genetic weakness, where the genes are mutated; in such a case, inside that cell there is a genetic 'time bomb' in which certain genes are triggered by some outside influence to begin to attack and corrode the cell nucleus where the gene pool is. Where we carry an inheritance of a weak genetic pool or contaminated gene material (e.g. the mother may have had diabetes) the genes will be carrying certain specific chemical messages which make those cells weak, with poor wall structure and not properly differentiated.

Every cell contains a specific matrix containing a printout for a specific form; each will be destined to become a particular cell in the body, and each chromosome has its own memory gene and knows exactly where to go. But in cell damage there is a gene explosion, e.g. when toxins cut across a cell leaving a chaotic array of genetic material which 'wants' to become a cell. Perhaps a cell that is destined normally to be part of the lung arrives in the liver; mutated cells will grow wherever they end up, even though they bear no relationship to other cells around them, a colony of these 'incorrect' cells gradually building up status inside tissue where they do not belong.

If someone lives at a high level of stress that is unresolved, the stress accentuates the level of carcinogenic secretions that are produced in the metabolism, plus perhaps alien microorganisms (like yeast) that get into the cell (easy once wounded and open to infiltration by any other toxins or oxidation). If this occurs, then the external toxic agents (e.g. through smoking) will be able to infiltrate the cells and gradually make inroads and weaken the nuclei. And once the nucleus is weakened, bits of genetic material can ooze out, every part of this genetic material 'wanting' to become a cell in its turn – and that means proliferation of mutated genes on their way to malignancy. It is a law of life that as soon as there is even a bit of a gene, every mutated piece 'wants' to become a cell and to become a nucleus – but it would do so without the full genetic information required for a cell to reach differentiation and maturity.

Perhaps the best way to fight stress is to find something absorbing to do and think about, preferably in the company of others with similar interests. You cannot think of two different things at once and complete concentration on, say, some form of art, meditation or any absorbing hobby will drive the worries out of your mind. If you can combine that with laughter, then your worries are reduced to such an extent that they no longer have adverse physical effects on you. As the editors of *Prevention* magazine said in their booklet *How to Boost Your Brain Power to Enrich Your Life*, 'He who laughs – lasts.'

5
WARNING SIGNS OF POTENTIAL CANCER

The following are some of the symptoms that have been frequently found in people who have developed cancer. Any one or more should not be taken as an indication that cancer will ensue, only that extra care should be taken to alter one's lifestyle so that the cancerous process is not helped in any way.

- Deficiencies of B vitamins, resulting in:
    Very red tongue.
    Cracks in corners of mouth and scaly circles around sides of nose.
    Dry and dead looking hair.
    Oedema on insides of lower legs, which are also sensitive to touch.
- Digestive diseases resulting in:
    Tremendous increase in alimentary gas or wind.
    Deficiency of pancreatic enzymes and stomach acidity, both giving wind.
    Burning sensation in one or more parts of the body due to sodium hydroxide irritation, but the affected place feels cold to the touch.
    Burning sensation in anus on bowel movement.
    Generally constipated.
- Unnatural blood conditions:
    High alkalinity or high acidity.
    Anaemia.
    Imbalance of proteins.
- Mental depression, when morbid thoughts creep into the mind:
    Apathy, listlessness, low vitality.
    Increased fatigue without real cause.
    Recurring thoughts of relatives who died from the disease.
- Sundry ailments that forecast degenerative diseases may be on their

way, but do NOT always, or even often, lead to cancer:
  Colitis, being overweight, emaciation.
  Rheumatism, arthritis.
  Bad circulation, varicose veins, cold hands and feet.
  Flu, liability to common cold, cold sores.
  Acne, eczema, psoriasis, dandruff, loss of hair.
  Sick headaches, hay fever, goitre.
  Angina.

- Toxic condition due to early childhood illnesses such as acne, styes, boils, mucus discharges, skin rashes, nausea, vomiting and fever, all of which are likely to have been due to excessive toxins in the system which the liver may not have been able to handle. Young adult women with menstrual problems are liable to have a toxic condition of the body; the toxins are 'dumped' in the uterus, which then becomes the seat of infection. If the uterus is removed, the toxins gravitate elsewhere and set up the conditions for cancer in a new place. (Note that a metallic odour from the womb is the first sign of cancer there.) At the menopause the escape route for toxins via the uterus is blocked and gives rise to illnesses such as hot flushes, nervous breakdowns, headaches, arthritis, neuritis, palpitations, vaginal discharges and ultimately malignancy may evolve.

- Sundry symptoms:
  Weakness in sight.
  Muscle aches in back and chest.
  Losing strength; losing hair, which becomes grey and brittle.
  Pain with deep breathing, plus high temperature.
  Muscle cramps of hands, feet or calves, usually when patient is about to fall asleep.
  Appearance of horny scales on skin.
  Bleeding of gums when teeth are brushed.
  Easy bruising.
  Loss of appetite and weight.
  Swelling of lymphatic glands: those on the left side of the neck may be diseased as a result of cancer of the gastrointestinal tract; those in the axilla (armpit) the result of cancer of the breast; those just above clavicle and beneath insertion of sternomastoid (the base of the neck, at the front) may mean bronchial carcinoma.
  Pigmentation of skin round umbilicus and anus, under breasts and in axillae may mean cancer of the intestines.

It should go without saying that the appearance of any of the above does not mean that cancer will develop, merely that these symptoms have appeared during the degenerative process.

Some extra signs of cancer:

- A burning pain with the passage of motion of the bowels, due to the unusual amount of sodium alkali in the faeces. The anal region too will feel as if burning.
- Excessive need for salt.
- Sciatica.
- High alkalinity of blood, with abnormal blueness of litmus paper test.
- Weak pulse, or increased in rate.
- Urine frequently alkaline.

Potential cancer patients often show some of the following characteristics, but people with these characteristics will not necessarily contract cancer.

- They may find it difficult to make close relationships, or perhaps only make one and if that ends there is a tremendous gap in their lives.
- Following on from this, they are often unable to show their feelings, either of affection or anger.
- This inability to show feelings may have grown up as a result of emotional starvation during their childhood; possibly they had reserved parents who did not themselves openly show emotion or affection towards their children.
- They may be rigid and perfectionists or, on the other hand, have a feeling of worthlessness.

CAN ONE TELL THE DIFFERENCE BETWEEN A MALIGNANT AND A BENIGN TUMOUR?

Unfortunately, not from its appearance. In a malignant tumour activity goes on inside the casing of the tumour which contravenes normal cellular order, i.e. a nest of fungal toxins may grow. As fungal organisms die back, the body tries to dialyse (get rid of) them, but if there is too much influx of inert material which gets stuck in a portion of the lymphatic system, the fungal toxins will 'nest' around, causing malignant changes in the cells.

Tumours will remain benign as long as there is not much carcinogenic activity but if there are a lot of activators around, then they will become malignant. And if the toxins get inside the genetic package in the cells, in other words if there is not just cell damage or oxidation but actual damage to the genetic material, then there will be an even greater chance of a malignant process setting in.

Simple microorganisms, such as staphylococci, will be content to perforate the cell wall, digest the cell plasma only and not interfere with the cell's nucleus. Those microorganisms however that do infiltrate into the nuclei, or chemicals like aluminium, lead, CO_2, which actually force their way into the nucleus, cause the genetic core to open up and many new 'rogue' cells are formed, resulting in the production of aggressive and tissue-damage-producing free radicals.

6
WHEN CANCER IS DIAGNOSED

- In most cases the patient and his or her family will be told; this will however be dependent on the mental state of the patient. Generally a counsellor who has been specially trained in helping patients through such crises will be able to reassure and answer the inevitable agonising questions.
- Join a cancer self-help group, where it is possible to talk openly with others who have been through the same experience.
- Realise that cancer patients are always under pressure from the medical authorities, from partners, parents and friends. But the ultimate decision on treatment lies with the patient.
- Read inspirational books by other sufferers. This will help to fight it, mentally.
- Check any negative feelings which may have been the cause of, or at least exacerbated, the symptoms. Review any emotional stresses over the preceding two years which may have triggered off the destructive process and led to the weakening of the immune system.
- Immediately start on Bach flower remedies − rock rose for panic, white chestnut for persistent worry, star of Bethlehem for after-effects of serious news, sweet chestnut for absolute dejection.
- Learn about what can and what cannot be eaten safely. What foods will increase the growth of the wrong intestinal flora and should therefore be avoided. Learn about the balancing of the intestinal flora, supplements to take to get rid of the wrong organisms (e.g. fluconazole, nystatin, Capricin) and how to restore the beneficial bacteria with acidophilus, bifidus supplementation or piima yoghourt. Learn about food combining.
- Learn about detoxification methods.
- Learn relaxation and visualisation, gentle exercise techniques, meridian massage, etc.
- Investigate methods of treatment other than suppressive, chemical or surgical.
- Realise that many cancers can be cured, but they all require a

maximum effort from the person concerned and a determination to overcome them. This is the reason why people with cancer *must* be told, so that they can face it themselves.

TREATMENT BY CHEMOTHERAPY

Once cancer has been diagnosed, conventional chemotherapy may be the only treatment considered possibly helpful. Chemotherapy places great demands on the body, however, so while it is being carried out, and afterwards, it is useful to consider how it may be possible to help the body cope with what is a great shock and stress to the system.

If the immune system is already low, chemotherapy will alter the balance of bacteria and yeasts in the small intestines and encourage the growth of unwanted bacteria and the proliferation of the yeast candida species, resulting in digestive problems. These problems may also result from a reduction in digestive enzyme production (the main symptom of which is wind after a meal), so supplementation may be required, or a change over to the Hay system of food combining (see Chapter 24).

Furthermore, although one's diet may be potentially healthy it is important to ensure that the nutrients in the food actually reach the tissues. Again, any problems in this field may be attributable to candida species and other organisms which can form a pseudo-wall of micellium clusters in the intestine walls, preventing nutrients from passing through into the bloodstream.

Some people find they need more protein than normal while undergoing chemotherapy, so it will not be possible to undertake complete detoxification programmes while on chemotherapy. Chemotherapy treatment may also involve the use of steroids, which may unbalance the blood sugar levels; it is then important to avoid all sugar in the diet and have frequent small meals.

Homoeopathic nosodes of the substances being used in the chemotherapy may help to counter their side effects. Other homoeopathic remedies, based on the principle of like curing like, will help. Homoeopathic first aid remedies, such as ipec or nux vomica for nausea, may be very useful during chemotherapy, while rescue remedy or other Bach flower remedies may help overcome the fear and panic associated with this treatment.

Visualisation and imagery (see Chapter 31) can be a great help in reinforcing the treatment and to form defences against the harmful effects of the chemotherapy.

Everyone in hospital has the right to ask for a healer to visit them –

all methods of healing, conventional or otherwise, are merely devices to gain time and to put the body into a state in which it can heal itself.

7
PREVENTION OF CANCER

Steps to take to minimise the chances of getting cancer, either for the first time or as a recurrence of a previous malignancy, fall into a number of categories:

- Better nutrition
- Stimulation of the immune system
- Stress prevention and management
- Lifestyle improvements
- Lastly, but by no means the least important, the will to live a creative life.

NUTRITION

If one assumes that one is in a precancerous state, without being morbid about it, it is merely commonsense to eat the things that help and avoid those that can harm someone who is not 100 per cent fit. It will therefore be necessary:

- To eat the right foods in the right combinations. This is clearly outlined in books dealing with the Hay diet (see Chapter 24).
- To plan the day's eating in such a way as to allow sufficient time and energy to eliminate the food residues and waste products which otherwise would pile up and ferment, thus providing an ideal breeding ground for candida and other microorganisms which would eventually lead to cancer or some other degenerative disease. (This is a major concept in the book *Fit for Life* by Harvey and Marilyn Diamond.)
- To eat foods to assist in the elimination process, i.e. eat sufficient healthy fibre, which helps to neutralise carcinogenic substances in various ways. It accelerates intestinal transit of food products, thus reducing the time that toxic substances are in contact with the intestinal walls and reducing the chances of a pile up of fermenting waste matter in the intestines. Studies have shown that people on a

low-fibre diet are three times more likely to get cancer than those on a high-fibre diet; there appears to be a link between low-fibre diets and lung cancer in particular. The fibre also 'fixes' carcinogenic materials in the intestinal tract, thus helping in their elimination in the stools. And finally, fibre reduces the absorption of fatty matter by incorporating it in the faeces (an excess of fatty substances is one of the factors favouring cancer).

- To eat foods which help in mopping up free radicals. Foods such as avocados, persimmons, papaya, kiwi fruit and some greens are all good in this regard.

- To choose foods which are full of anticarcinogenic substances and contain fibre, chlorophyll, vitamin E, selenium and some indoles and phenols as are found in green vegetables, primarily the cabbage family, and in particular broccoli and brussels sprouts. These are rich in vitamin C, indoles and fibre, as well as other protective elements.

- To find foods which are rich in beta-carotene which is an antioxidant and free radical blocker. One of the principal sources is, of course, carrots, but it is also in cabbages, broccoli, salsify, cress, lambs' lettuce, spinach, marrow, courgettes, pumpkins (rich in vitamin C, carotenoids and fibre), red beetroot, water cress, swedes (the leaves more than the roots), petit pois. (It is unfortunate that very small young vegetables, e.g. green beans, peas, courgettes, have a higher level of nitrates if picked at that stage and are poorer in fibre and vitamins – gourmet chefs please note.)

- To have foods which have been lacto-fermented (fermented by whey), which are said to be both preventative and curative of cancers. Lactic acid has a positive effect on cell respiration, which would normally be slowed down in cancerous cells.

- To eat foods which are right for you. Coeliacs, for instance, cannot tolerate gluten; if they have glutenous foods they damage the mucosa of the lining of the small intestine, making it more permeable to cancer-causing toxins. A lack of vitamin A can also increase the risk of cancer in coeliacs.

- Always try and find foods which are organically grown. They contain less nitrates than chemically grown ones and their loss of vitamins is negligible if consumed fresh.

STIMULATION OF THE IMMUNE SYSTEM

Cancer is a disease of the whole organism, even though it may appear in only one place at first. It is therefore the whole body which needs treatment. Cutting out the offending organ will only be fully successful in those cases where the act of cutting out the focus of disease will allow the body time to fight it in other parts before it manifests itself again.

Stimulation of the protective system of the body will include:

- Vitamin and mineral supplementation.
- Strengthening of the bodily tissues (collagen) with vitamin C and bioflavonoids.
- Pancreatic enzyme supplementation.
- Plant extracts such as Iscador (mistletoe extract), Abnova Viscum.
- Detoxification of the body.

STRESS PREVENTION

Dr Contreras of the Centro Medico del Mar in Mexico, a cancer specialist known the world over, contends that as high as 75 per cent of cancers could be due to excessive stress. It is difficult to disagree with this hypothesis when one thinks about one's friends who have contracted cancer. Many will have been living apparently healthy lives, eating organically grown food, not smoking or drinking, doing a normal amount of exercise, and yet they got cancer. But if one delves, one can usually find stresses which have been bottled up, or even stresses which the individual did not appreciate as being long-term stresses, such as the death of a close relative. Life crises and unfinished business in our emotional make-up need attention.

LIFESTYLE

Under this heading one can include geographic factors. In a study carried out by the Medical Research Council and documented in 1984 in the *Atlas of Cancer Mortality in England and Wales* (published by John Wiley), certain cancers were conspicuous in certain areas. Some were caused from purely environmental influences, like nasal cancer in people working in the furniture-making trade and lung cancer caused through asbestos dust. On the other hand, cancers such as stomach cancer, which is numerically highest in Wales, may be attributed to diets deficient in fresh foods. Women who have a number of children at a young age are less likely to get breast cancer than those who start a family later in life.

At the time of the report, Britain had the highest proportion of reported deaths from lung cancer of any country in the world. There seems to be no doubt whatever that this is linked to smoking. Anyone who smokes is putting him or herself at risk unnecessarily – the statistics are too overwhelming. The conclusion has to be that, a smoker is showing, perhaps unknowingly, a decreased will to live.

Exercise on a regular basis can be beneficial in strengthening organs:

- It reduces high blood pressure.
- It strengthens the heart and lungs.
- It reduces the chance of heart attacks.
- It reduces blood glucose levels.
- It reduces the loss of calcium from bones (osteoporosis).
- It relieves stress, which is a great enemy of a healthy immune system.
- It increases levels of endorphins, the brain hormones that create a feeling of well-being.

But excessive exercise can be harmful, particularly if not accompanied by proper nutrition, and particularly in certain diseases like ME; moderation should be the keyword. Warm-up exercises – stretching – are good, then finishing with cooling down exercise to help the circulation return to normal.

Laughter can be a potent aid in recovery and prevention. It has been said that no really happy person gets cancer. Gatherings of patients and friends at Springhill are notable for their happy atmosphere; a stranger who dropped in the middle of a teaching session there could be excused if he thought the members of the group were old friends out on a day's trip in the country. Laughter promotes a healing atmosphere and, through the friendships established in such gatherings, a new and improved quality of life sets in. This is in stark contrast to the atmosphere in most hospital waiting rooms, where fear is positively tangible and any conversations are carried out in hushed tones as if the participants were in church. A notable example of the power of laughter is recounted in the book *Anatomy of an Illness* by Norman Cousins (Penguin Books).

THE WILL TO LIVE

This is a potent factor in the rehabilitation and cure of people with life-threatening diseases. The strength of a person's will to live can be judged by their actions. Perhaps a woman does not consider it necessary to be screened for possible breast cancer regularly, despite the fact that this process can cut the incidence of breast cancers by a third. Anyone who smokes heavily is consciously defying the statistical evidence of the connection of smoking with lung and other cancers and, unconsciously, is showing a fatalistic unconcern over the probable length of their life.

As part of a programme for taking control of one's own health one should study the literature devoted to complementary methods of treatment, and discuss with fellow sufferers treatments that they have found helpful. It is amazing how ignorant most of us are about the workings of our own bodies and minds and this can be a fascinating study, with a very worthwhile aim and priceless rewards.

Everyone needs to participate in their own cancer prevention and rehabilitation and not follow a lifestyle that they know is dangerous to their health.

PREVENTING THE RECURRENCE OF DISEASE

Operations, even if successful, leave the patient anxious as to whether cancer will reappear, perhaps in some other part of the body. The only way to overcome this fear is to work to increase the immune system's power to destroy cancer cells. It is possible for cancer to be present in the body and yet for the body to be in control of it, but all cancer patients fear the possibility of recurrence and are continually looking for signs of such a thing happening. Minor aches and pains assume a significance out of all proportion to their actual distress.

Any change in a person's condition for the better will normally take some time, and there may be temporary ups and downs. Recognition of any change, for the better or for the worse, is useful feedback for helping a person take further positive steps towards recovery. For example, it is useful to be prepared for a temporary worsening of symptoms, and to realise that this *is* probably only a temporary phase. The recurrence should then perhaps be used to re-examine the reasons behind the illness and why it might recur:

- Have you given in to an emotional conflict?
- Is the illness being used to resolve some emotional conflicts? Review the unconsciously desired 'benefits' you may be expecting from the illness.
- Are you trying to change things too fast? This is in itself a form of stress.
- Have you given up the healthy regime, physical or mental, which in the first place produced some improvement, possibly because of complacency once its benefits were felt?

Critically examine what might be the reasons behind the recurrence, and if necessary make changes in thought or action. The aim should clearly be to do everything possible to make one's body as healthy as possible, to build up one's immune system, so that it can resist any further carcinogens on the move. It is not, however, sufficient just to do without obvious cancer-forming substances or to give up habits such as smoking: there will be psychological, mental and emotional pressures as well, any of which may be nurturing the cancer.

Emotions should be expressed; the mere fact of not losing one's temper does not mean one is not angry, it only means that the anger gets bottled up and comes out as some form of disease. Suppressed emotions can cause a lot of physical as well as mental problems, through the build-up of stress, leading to tension and physical ailments.

8
THE IMMUNE SYSTEM

Before we look in detail at the immune system, let us first look at the invading organisms and toxins with which it has to deal.

An antigen is a general term for a foreign substance that invades the body – bacteria, viruses, fungi, dust, harmful chemicals and pollutants, pollen grains, proteins from food that hasn't been properly digested, etc. These antigens are recognised by specific receptors within the immune system and thereby trigger the system into action; specific antibodies are produced against the antigen, neutralising it; the cells of the immune system swing into action, engulfing it. It is the specific pattern of the antigen and its chemical constituents that the immune system locks on to and against which it mounts a specific attack.

Antigens may have been introduced deliberately into the body, perhaps in the form of organ transplants or through blood transfusions of an incompatible blood type, in which case the immune system's normal response may cause unpleasant reactions. This fact makes necessary the use of immune system suppressive (immunosuppressive) drugs in transplant surgery; however, these drugs so depress the immune system that it cannot cope with other serious, and therefore often fatal, illnesses.

Antigens may also originate within the body, such as cancer cells. In a healthy body they are recognised and attacked before they have the chance to grow out of control.

Antigens are mostly protein. For example, they occur on many sites (antigenic sites) on the shell of a virus or the cell wall of a bacterium. The immune system has the ability to recognise and retaliate against several million antigens. If it has not previously met an antigen, this reaction will take time, and if the immune system has been weakened the body may not be able to react sufficiently in time.

VIRUSES

A virus is a protein-coated bundle of genetic material (DNA or RNA) containing built-in instructions for replicating (making copies of itself).

Viruses are extremely minute – far smaller than a living cell – and can only be seen with the aid of a high-magnification electron microscope. Viruses either enter the cells of their particular target host cell or inject their genetic material, the protein shell being discarded. The viral genes (the DNA or RNA) then take over the host cell and get it to make replicas of the virus in large numbers in a very short time – even as short a time as 20 minutes – at the same time suppressing the cell's normal functions. Great quantities of viruses are produced until eventually the cell cannot hold them, ruptures and dies, and the many viruses move on to repeat the process. Through the damage done to the host cells the way may be open to secondary infection by bacteria (which are comparatively large organisms about 100 to 200 times the size of viruses, and visible through a good optical microscope).

Viruses thus cannot reproduce on their own and have to use cells of the body to help them. Indeed, they may cause their host cells to produce further infected cells, which thus shield the virus from the body's defences. Viruses are:

- Kept in check by antibodies (immunoglobulins) which may kill virus-infected cells.
- Can be killed through the action of the cells of the immune system, aided by the lymphokines such as interferon, interleukins and other immune cell behaviour modifiers.
- Research indicates that vitamin C in high doses (even up to bowel tolerance dose) has been found useful in destroying viruses.
- Antibiotics do not kill viruses; they only affect bacteria.

Viral diseases include colds, flu, measles, German measles, rabies, smallpox, mumps, hepatitis types A and B, herpes, HIV and a number of the malignant and severely disabling diseases like MS or motor neurone disease.

RETROVIRUSES

Some viruses link up their genetic material with that of the host cell. These are called retroviruses and may remain quiescent in the host cell for varying periods until they are induced (triggered) into action and replication by such things as ultraviolet or X-ray radiation. This results in a proliferation of faulty cells and in the eventual death of the host cells. There is then a chain reaction in the production of faulty cells and the faulty genetic knowledge becomes part of these faulty cells' genetic structure. There is growing evidence of a link between retroviruses and cancers, leukaemias, lymphomas and other obscure diseases.

BACTERIA

Bacteria constitute an enormous group of microorganisms. Unlike viruses, they are complete living organisms that can survive and flourish outside a host cell. However, not only can pathogenic bacteria flourish on or in us, compromising the effectiveness of the tissues or organs they have invaded, but they can also produce toxins – poisons – which can have wide-ranging effects on the whole organism.

The immune system attacks bacteria in a similar way to that with which it deals with viruses:

- Antibodies are secreted, and attach themselves to the surface of the bacteria, thereby damaging them.
- The bacteria can be gobbled up by some cells of the immune system.
- Another group of immune system cells releases enzymes and other chemicals that destroy the bacteria.
- The toxins produced by the bacteria can be neutralised by antibodies.

Amid all this immune system activity, some innocent tissue can get caught up and damaged, giving rise to an abscess. Or, on a wider scale, a fever may result. Fevers are part of our natural defence system – most microorganisms are destroyed by heat. Rest and plenty of fluids are important for a therapeutic antifever routine.

Because bacteria can be controlled and destroyed by antibiotics, the major bacterial diseases such as diphtheria, whooping cough, typhoid, tuberculosis, botulism, and tetanus are not nearly as common now as they were, say, 50 years ago; vaccinations and inoculations have also had an important impact. But these 'advances' have encouraged more pathogenic strains of bacteria that were previously relatively innocuous to develop – for example the organisms that cause boils and sore throats.

WHAT IS THE IMMUNE SYSTEM?

The immune system is the first line of defence the body has against toxic and viral, bacterial or fungal attack and it responds in each individual in an identical way to all disease, regardless of its cause or where in the body the disease is. It has the responsibility for:

- Recognising toxic substances which are attacking the body's cells.
- Overcoming such attacks.

It has the capacity to recognise and deal with 'foreign' substances but can 'tolerate' substances belonging to the body. Any substances that are foreign to the body are recognised by the cells of the lymph system; the immune system then gets to work to isolate the trouble and prevent it from spreading.

Vaccinations (or immunisations) are a method of giving the body a weakened, or dead, strain of virus or bacteria so that it will recognise a similar pathogen again and have the necessary defences (antibodies) ready for quick action. Vaccinations may, however, bring very serious side effects and, particularly in the case of measles, have been seen as being the cause of many serious diseases, including brain damage, seizures, childhood leukaemias and possibly SIDS (sudden infant death syndrome, or 'cot deaths'). Metabolic mistakes and faulty genetic make-up are common with some forms of vaccination. Diseases resulting from vaccinations come under the heading of vaccinosis.

The immune system is a very flexible system and can adapt itself to fight different forms of pathogens (organisms that produce disease) such as viruses, bacteria, moulds, as well as chemicals, etc., etc.

The body's defences include:

- The skin, including the acidic sweat.
- The mucous membranes of the respiratory system (easily damaged by smoking).
- The mucous membranes of the digestive system.
- The acidity of the stomach, although this may be bypassed by pathogens in any undigested food that gets into the intestines.
- Lysozyme, an enzyme in tears.
- B and T cells of the immune system.
- Glycoproteins of the immune system, which surround microorganisms, so stopping them from reaching their target cells.

The presence of pathogens does not necessarily imply that a person will get ill. This only happens if there is a weakness in the immune defensive system.

Immune deficiency diseases may be genetic, i.e. inherited. The immune system efficiency may be impaired further as a result of factors such as aging, stress, malnutrition, immunosuppressant drugs, malignancies, excess radiation (including sunlight) or as a result of diseases such as AIDS, where the body suppresses the immune functions.

Immunosuppressants include:

- Radiation, even low level radiation such as medical X-rays, radioactive materials, exposure to leaking microwaves, all of which are higher than normal background sources, and whose effects on the body tend to accumulate. Foetuses particularly may be affected, and infantile cancers often result when the mother has been exposed to these hazards during pregnancy.

- Ultraviolet radiation in sunlight suppresses the immune system response and can result in skin problems and skin cancers. The body is even more sensitive to these radiations if cortisone is being used for some reason (e.g. on eczemas) or when toxic compounds are being used to pigment the skin, such as rancid oils or psoralens.
- Immunosuppressive drugs, e.g. used to prevent graft rejection.
- Sex hormone alternatives (e.g. the pill, steroids, medication).
- Stress.
- Malnutrition.
- Alcohol.
- Numerous viruses, bacteria and fungi.

Those genetically predisposed – people whose families show one or more cancers – need to be particularly careful to avoid contact with carcinogens, as their immune system is probably not strong enough to defend them against such immune-depressing agents.

The active constituents of the immune system consists of white blood cells, lymph cells, antibodies, compounds known as complement and interferon, and other non-specific antimicrobial serum factors. These circulate in the bloodstream and, more importantly, in the lymphatic system.

The lymphatic system:

- Protects against infection and disease.
- Carries nutrients to every cell in the body.
- Is made up of primary and secondary organs, and circulatory vessels, similar to the veins of the blood system.

The primary organs are where the protective cells are produced, such as the thymus gland and bone marrow. The thymus gland in particular is responsible for the development of the body's immune system, and shrinks rapidly under stress – demonstrating the body's needs for it. Science thought for years that the thymus wasted after puberty and had no *raison d'être* after that age; it was noticed, in post mortems on dead bodies, that the thymus totally calcified after puberty and was entirely covered by a thick membrane of mucus surrounded by fibrous, hardened and very tough tissue. Therefore it was assumed it could not act as a gland. It is now known that our immunity depends entirely on the production of a certain hormone called thymoxin, produced by the thymus, which goes to 'imprint' our protective T cells (see below). We do not produce T cells if the thymus is not working. If a child develops infections, particularly recurrent ones, it is because the thymus is not producing T cells and the body cannot therefore fight infections. Gradual atrophy of the thymus gland leaves the person short of his protective T cells.

The secondary organs, i.e. the lymph nodes, spleen, tonsils, appendix, Peyers patches (sites of small glands in the small intestines), are where the battle between foreign substances and the defence system takes place.

The lymph nodes are knots of cells on the lymphatic vessels, that filter the lymph in order to protect a particular part of the body, e.g. nodes on the neck protect the head, those at the top of the thighs protect the legs and genitals, etc. These lymph nodes become enlarged as a result of any infection and are a sign that the body is taking action to try to fend off invaders.

The body's circulating defence system consists mainly of white cells or leucocytes of the blood; these cells make up less than 1 per cent of the total cells in the blood, the remainder being red blood cells, whose function is the transport of oxygen. About 25 per cent of these leucocytes are called lymphocytes, so-called because they are very plentiful in the lymph and are concentrated in lymph nodes, ready to fight infection.

LYMPHOCYTES

Lymphocytes are divided into two groups.

T cells (thymus derived lymphocytes) originate in the stem cells in bone marrow, but are 'imprinted' in their millions by the thymus gland's hormones. They circulate through the body and are made up of four major kinds.

- Inducer or helper-T cells have the task of alerting other cells and guiding them in to the attack; these helper cells release interleukins, which take messages from lymphocyte to lymphocyte.
- The second group, once alerted by the helper-T cells, release enzymes around any foreign material, and these enzymes in turn activate the macrophages that engulf the antigen or that release harmful chemicals that neutralise it.
- Killer-T cells are 'instructed' by the interleukins released by the helper cells to attach themselves to the foreign invader. They then, like the macrophages, release chemicals which neutralise and destroy it.

- The last group are regulatory T cells. These limit the range and scope of the immune response by the other T cells to an appropriate level. Without these cells an immune response might overwhelm the body as well as the invader. These are the T-suppressor cells.

In AIDS the HIV virus invades the T-helper cells and eventually knocks them out, thus removing an important link in the chain of the immune response.

The second group of lymphocytes are the B cells, so called because they mature in the bone marrow. Like the T cells, each B cell is programmed to react to one, and only one, of a huge range of antigens. A neighbouring B cell will react with another antigen, and so on, so that the entire range of antigens that the body might have to face is covered.

The B cells live in the lymph nodes, but only survive for a few weeks; consequently the bone marrow is continuously producing them.

- If a specific antigen comes along and is recognised by the appropriate B cell, the B cell is then activated by a T-helper cell.
- The activated B cell then starts to manufacture proteins called antibodies, these antibodies being specific to the antigen. The antibodies help destroy the antigen through combining with the chemical marker on the antigen.
- The specific B cells involved in this reaction are subsequently responsible for storing the memory of the antigen (the process being called an anamnestic response). Thus the body has a rapid response to antigens it has met in the past. (This is the principle of immunisation and vaccination.)
- Once activated, the B cells 'clone' themselves in large numbers to produce specific antibodies, as and when required, to fight off their particular antigen. After an infectious illness, therefore, the body retains an acquired immunity for some time (a 'memory'), the period differing for different diseases.
- The activated B cells that are producing antibodies are often referred to as plasma cells. They can, very quickly, manufacture huge quantities of antibodies specific to the antigen which caused the production of the antibody – they are factories for the production of antibody, which sticks to the surface of the invading viruses, bacteria, fungi, protozoa, or whatever, damaging them and making them easier targets for the granulocytes to devour and destroy.

MACROPHAGES

Once the T cells have been activated they release enzymes that attract the macrophages. The macrophages are large cells that engulf the antigen that the T cells have recognised – perhaps a virus or bacteria – and then destroy the antigen once it is inside the macrophage's cell membrane. Alternatively they release chemicals that inactivate and neutralise the antigen.

The macrophages are produced in the bone marrow and released in an immature form known as monocytes. They circulate in the blood-stream and lymphatic system, or reside in the ducts and channels of the organs of the lymphatic system. Once called into action by the T cells the monocytes rapidly mature into macrophages.

Macrophages are particularly useful in fighting tumours, viral, fungal and bacterial infections, but in doing so they produce free radicals (see Chapter 17).

GRANULOCYTE/POLYMORPHONUCLEAR CELLS

Once antibodies have been released by the B cells, after challenge from an antigen and activation by the helper T cells, the antibodies attach themselves to the antigens, as we have seen.

They also bring into action what is known as the complement system. The complement system is a series of chemicals that normally circulates in the blood lymph, perfectly innocuously. But once brought into action by the antibodies, the complement system is transformed into a chain reaction that homes in on the antigen alongside the anti-bodies. And some elements of this complement chain reaction call into play the granulocytes or polymorphonuclear cells.

These cells act in a similar way to the macrophages, i.e. they engulf or swallow up antigens, but only antigens – principally bacteria – that are coated with antibody and complement. The granulocytes are there-fore a key group of cells if the B-cell system is to function properly.

KILLER AND NATURAL KILLER CELLS

This last group of leucocytes in some ways resembles B and T cells to look at, but its actions are distinct.

- The killer cells, or K cells, attack foreign cells that have been coated with antibody. They appear to be important in our defence against cancer.
- Natural killer or NK cells appear to be able to destroy certain cells and

invading organisms without any assistance from any other branches of the immune system, although they do seem to work more efficiently in the presence of chemicals released by activated T cells.

ANTIBODIES

Antibodies, as we have seen, are produced by the B lymphocytes of the immune system, although a new-born baby will have acquired a protective range of antibodies across the placenta or through the colostrum of the mother's milk. Natural immunity therefore starts at or before birth. After that, antibodies are produced by the B cells in direct response to the presence of antigens, reacting specifically with those antigens.

There appears to be no limit to the number of different antibodies a person's immune system can produce, and virtually every foreign protein which invades a body will cause a unique antibody to be formed, specifically matched with the antigen. Some are acquired through necessity as a result of attack by foreign substances, while others can be acquired passively through introduction of antibodies extracted from a person who has already had the disease (or been vaccinated against it). The first time our immune defences are challenged by an antigen, say measles virus, it takes about 14 days for the B-cell system to swing into action and to produce enough antibodies to cope with the infection. However, once the B-cell system has been primed in this way it takes a much shorter time to cope with a subsequent challenge by the same antigen.

As we have seen, antibodies stick to the surface of invading viruses, bacteria, fungi, and protozoa, damaging them and making them easier targets for the granulocytes to devour and destroy.

Antibodies occur in five major groups, but all consist of proteins known as immunoglobulins. Each immunoglobulin (IgG) consists of Y-shaped molecules, the top half of which constitutes the specific receptor for a specific antigen. If the Y-shaped top of the antibody makes contact with its appropriate antigen, it locks itself firmly on, causing the invader to become coated with antibody molecules and thereby making it more vulnerable to phagocytosis.

IgG is the major antibody that coats microorganisms to make them more palatable and speed their uptake by the scavenging immune cells. IgG levels may be increased by coenzyme Q10 (possibly taking 2–3 months at a daily rate of 60 mg of CoQ10).

COMPLEMENT

As we have seen, complement is a series of 11 different chemicals, all of which must be present for it to have any effect. Complement molecules congregate round the antibody, and help bind together antigen and antibody. These three substances then form a macromolecule called an immune complex, which is normally destroyed by the granulocytes.

INTERFERON

Interferon is a chemical messenger released by T cells. It stops protein manufacture by cells invaded by viruses only, so that the virus cannot increase in number. It also helps cells not yet infected to resist the virus. It is now recognised as a first line of defence; it is a non-specific anti-viral protein. This interferon does not directly attack the viruses, but makes contact with surrounding healthy cells, and, through liberation of another protein, makes them less susceptible to the virus, which is then unable to use those cells to replicate. The white cells can then dispose of any dead cell debris.

Interferon also seems to stimulate NK cells to kill virus-infected and malignant cells. Many patients who suffer from depression have abnormally low levels of NK cells, perhaps due to poor production of interferon. Vitamin C can stimulate the production of interferon, and fevers improve the effectiveness of interferon.

INFLAMMATION AND FEVER

Inflammation and fever are induced by the release of histamine, and are defensive actions by the body (unless and until it becomes too extensive and thereby harmful). Put simply, the two processes increase the blood supply to a site of infection or antigenic invasion, so that it is well supplied with both lymphocytes and phagocytes.

Histamine and various other inflammatory chemicals are contained within mast cells, which are in turn liberally scattered around the body. Attached to the mast cells is a specialised variety of antibody, the tail of which is fixed to the mast cell membrane and the antigen receptor of which faces outwards. When an antigen locks on to the antibody on the mast cells the reaction causes the mast cell to explode, releasing the inflammatory chemicals, which in turn dilate the surrounding blood vessels and allow other elements of the immune system to squeeze through and attack the invader.

TOLERANCE

The immune system can recognise (or tolerate) parts of the body, as against substances that are foreign to it; it will ignore stimuli that originate within the body. This is not however always to the benefit of the individual as it may tolerate unwanted happenings in the body, such as tumour growths, unwittingly allowing them to grow. The obverse is the basis of autoimmune diseases, in which the body starts to react against, and disrupt, itself.

THE IMMUNE SYSTEM AND THE BRAIN

There is evidence that there is direct control of the immune system by the brain, either:

- Indirectly through hormones in the bloodstream; or
- Directly through the nerves and their neurochemical synthesis.

As all activities of cells in our bodies are under the control of the brain, consciously or not, it follows that the brain has to be supplied with the correct nutrients, via the blood, to keep it operating efficiently.

Instructions from the brain to cells and tissues are delivered by chemical messengers called neurotransmitters, secreted at nerve endings. The nervous system depends on these neurotransmitters for the rapid transmission of messages from one nerve cell to the next. The main neurotransmitters that affect the nervous system are:

- Acetylcholine, which also can activate B and T cell production and affects the thymus gland.
- Serotonin (5HT) which, on the other hand, inhibits the production of antibodies, i.e. it is an immunosuppressant, and can regulate the hypothalamus and pineal gland hormone throughput.
- Dopamine, which is a stimulant to the immune system and appears to reduce the effectiveness of the T-suppressor cells. A deficiency of dopamine has been shown in patients with Parkinson's disease.

These neurotransmitters can be boosted through an intake of specific amino acid precursors, either as part of one's diet, or by supplementation; the amount of each neurotransmitter in the brain will depend on the quantity and availability of the crucial amino acids. Careful monitoring of metabolic activity can enable the physician to ascertain which amino acids are required for corrective therapy. The key precursor:

- For acetylcholine is choline, as found in lecithin, fish, eggs, etc.

- For serotonin is tryptophan, found in many foods such as eggs, meat, fish, milk, flour, cheese, beans, peas, etc. A deficiency of tryptophan leads to less B lymphocyte production. Tryptophan requires vitamins B3, B6 and C to help it transform to serotonin. If tryptophan is being taken as an aid to sleep, then a carbohydrate meal should be taken last thing at night as this increases production of serotonin, which helps the uptake of other amino acids in the body tissues but not tryptophan. Then tryptophan is therefore left in the blood circulation and is free to pass through the blood/brain barrier while there is no competition from other amino acids.
- For dopamine is tyrosine, which stimulates production of noradrenaline which is a derivative of dopamine. Tyrosine is helpful as an antidepressant and stimulates a positive mental outlook, so is essential to the maintenance of a strong immune system.

To make the best use of amino acids it is better to have a low protein, high complex-carbohydrate diet, plus vitamins and minerals as appropriate to the condition.

The mind can affect the immune system through the chemical messages created by and sent by the brain. The hypothalamus (a small area in the brain) when under stress, triggers the pituitary gland which in turn causes the adrenal glands to release adrenaline and corticosteroids which prevent the immune system from responding normally to infections and other challenges. Corticosteroids are powerful immunosuppressants, and they have an influence on the evolution of many illnesses, including cancer.

The main factor which disrupts the brain's control is chronic stress, which actually encourages the adrenals to produce hormones as part of the 'fight or flight' response to the stress, and these hormones can suppress the immune system's responses. They also reduce the effect of interferon. Therefore a positive outlook can actually affect the body's physical response to viral attack. (Note that vitamin C is the safest substance to take to reduce the corticosteroids produced by over-stimulation of the adrenals.)

The state of mind therefore has an immediate and direct effect on the state of our body, which we can change, for better or worse, by the nature of the thoughts we have. Bereavement is well known to have a delayed action response, so that a major illness often strikes some 18 months to two years after a bereavement in the family. Our mental attitude can even affect how infectious diseases are coped with when our production of antibodies is faulty. It is thus a person's ability to cope with stress that is more important than the stress itself.

One needs to visualise the changes one wants in one's body through the feelings and emotions, which have a strong effect on the body's rhythms and workings. This may explain the healing powers of placebos, of faith healing, of meditation, of prayer, etc., all of which assume their use is leading to better health. Relaxation is also essential, i.e. you cannot be relaxed and stressed at the same time – as Emile Coue said, 'it is impossible to think of two things at once'. These techniques help a person to develop a positive expectancy about the outcome of their disease, particularly if the underlying causes are understood and positive steps are taken to correct them. This is in stark contrast with a person's normal concentration on the symptoms of, say, cancer (even though the cancer may in the end prove beneficial through having brought to the individual's notice the underlying problems in their lives).

Dr Edward Bach, who developed the Bach flower remedies, realised that negative states of mind weaken the body's inborn resistance to stress and disease and often poison the system, hindering the effectiveness of any treatment. His remarkable accounts and experiences with his flower extracts are well documented. It is therefore useful to check which of the 38 negative states of mind Bach identified are behind the weakness of a particular individual's immune system (see page 257).

THE IMMUNE SYSTEM AND AGING

T-cell shortages, following deterioration of the thymus gland, which starts at puberty, occur in aging people and result in reduced immunity. Gradually the production of thymoxin hormone gets less and less, so the T cells, which need it, become abnormal and allow toxins to attack and ravage the body. There is also a decline in coenzyme Q10 (an important cofactor in many chemical reactions in the body – see page 55) in proportion to the decreasing weight of the thymus gland. This results in a weakened immune system in old age; it then cannot produce adequate antibodies against an antigen, and results in a greater probability of diseases which are normally kept at bay.

Habitual lifelong adherence to a low-calorie diet (with adequate nutrients, vitamins and minerals) could prevent immune failure and sustain youthfulness. Such a diet helps to keep the thymus gland functional for a longer time, and also makes one more resistant to cancer, arthritis, heart and vascular disease, dementia and all the motor disorders.

One medical stratagem to reduce some of the problems of aging is to use T- and B-cell therapy. These cells are taken from a patient while his immune system is functioning normally and stored at a very low temperature. They are then reintroduced to the patient to restore the immune system to nearly normal competence and to increase lifespan.

CANCER AND THE IMMUNE SYSTEM

Cancer only appears when the immune system is not functioning properly, or when it has perhaps become suppressed and cannot deal with invading toxins. Therefore anything that upsets the brain's control of the immune system will increase the chance of malignancy. Even passive emotions such as grief, suppression of anger or feelings of failure mean an overproduction of the hormones which suppress the immune-system responses.

Alternatively, people with cancer may, in essence, have a strong immune system, but they overproduce the straightforward lymphocytes, macrophages, granulocytes, etc. People who have developed a degenerative disease of any kind all tend to overproduce these cells.

Tumours are a way of isolating cellular byproducts that the organism cannot assimilate. An encapsulated tumour has a life of its own separate from the life of the individual, plant or animal; it has no connection in its genetic memory with the organisation and processes of the rest of the body; it has its own life-regulating cycles. It is the result of the defensive action of the body. If one has blood, lymph, nerve, plasma or bone-marrow cancers, it means the body no longer has the capacity to encapsulate and isolate these malignant cells and toxins. In contrast, solid tumours are an indication that a person's immune system is still working and has been able to isolate the active toxins and microorganisms within the shell of the tumour. Note, however, that sometimes what looks like a tumour on an X-ray, while still being a cancer, may be in origin a nest of microorganisms (byproducts of candida, for example) that have proliferated and caused changes in the tissues. This may even occur in the bones, where the pain of cancer is the most severe. It might even be just an active candida nest; this would still show on a scan as a shadow suggesting a tumour. Only histological investigation which screens the tissues, not only for malignant neoplasia but for microorganisms, will give a true diagnosis.

It is for this reason that, by going on an exclusion programme and an antifungal diet, it is possible for 'tumours' to regress and the tissues to heal very rapidly, simply because the main trigger factors will have been removed. These 'tumours', if they are not given the necessary nutrients via the bloodstream, will dry up and cells will revert to their normal status.

In contrast, the immune system responses of the person with leukaemia or bone marrow cancer have diminished far more than a person with an encapsulated tumour. The potential for isolating a solid tumour, and then, once you have got rid of it, returning to positive health, is far greater in a person with an encapsulated tumour than someone with lymphoma (cancer in the lymph), neuroblastoma (cancer of the nervous system) or leukaemia (cancer of the blood). In those cancers that have no boundaries, no encapsulation, the immune system has obviously broken down; there will be concomitant active fungal and other microbial toxins which cannot be contained, i.e. kept in one place like a solid tumour, and they will be taken by the blood circulation to any weak organ or system.

NUTRITION AND THE IMMUNE SYSTEM

In malnutrition interferon production is inhibited, tonsils become shrunken, complement is reduced and metabolises incorrectly. Poor diets are short of essential amino acids and other necessary nutrients, which leads to decreased T-cell production and decreased phagocyte ability to destroy viruses, bacteria and fungi, making people more susceptible to viral, bacterial and fungal infections. There must therefore be adequate nutrition to give the immune system the nutrients it needs to protect the body. The following nutrients, supplements and suggestions are recommended for boosting or supporting the immune system.

- Vitamin C in large quantities, to tolerance levels. One of its functions is to form the collagen of connective tissues, and strong collagen fibres limit the passage of any viruses. Furthermore, daily doses of vitamin C increase the production of lymphocytes, which cancer patients have a poor ability to make.

- L-arginine, an amino acid, particularly recommended at the start of any anti-candida campaign helps the thymus gland to produce T cells (required as part of the immune-response system), but should not be given to anyone with a history of herpes, as it would exacerbate it.

- Increase the oxygen of the cells, as our immune system requires large quantities of oxygen to operate. This can be done by increasing the intake of germanium (found in garlic and *Aloe vera* particularly) which is also in mistletoe and may be the reason why Iscador has been beneficial in treating cancer (through the improvement in the immune system and specific changes in cell plasma as well as having selective cytotoxic properties against cancer cells).

- Coenzyme Q10 is a vital link in the metabolic machinery of living cells, stimulating mitochondria (which provide the energy for cellular function). A very great deal of energy is expended at cellular level, particularly when one is ill, in order to carry out the chemical reactions necessary for recovery, often leaving little energy for muscular action or possibly even for the action of the brain, confused through the many poisons in the blood. It has been suggested that supplementation with coenzyme Q10 will help restore the immune function and simultaneously forestall the aging process, and has been shown to be valuable in treating damaged heart muscle.

- Raw glandular products (animal glands that have been prepared as supplements at temperatures never exceeding normal body heat) have an affinity for the same gland and in fact encourage the activity of that particular gland. Also, homoeopathically potentised glandular tissue has now been used and documented in the specialist journals widely.

- By supplementation with yeast-free vitamins B6; B12 (folic acid); calcium pantothenate (vitamin B5), especially if there are any allergies (vitamin B can be given by injection, monthly); vitamin A as beta-carotene; vitamin F (evening primrose oil); vitamin E, vitamin C (buffered types) in megadoses to protect the body from acetaldehyde and other poisonous chemicals produced by candida and other micro-organisms

- Mineral supplementation with selenium; zinc orotate or citrate; magnesium orotate.

- Linseed oil for its linolenic acid which helps clear the intestines of fat and cholesterol and allows nutrients to be absorbed properly.

- Anything that will help to keep candida species in check, such as: vitamin C, buffered with calcium; Capricin, Mycoptyl, Diflucan or nystatin to kill candida, followed by live acidophilus and bifidus culture to replace the undesirable organisms in the intestines; biotin (vitamin B) to stop the yeast form of candida from turning into the more dangerous mycelial form; oleic acid from virgin olive oil (2 tsp in water twice a day); garlic (fresh or as capsules); *Aloe vera* juice (2 tsp in water twice a day); ginseng and pao d'arco tea infusion (two or three times daily).

- Nutrients to aid the production of corticosteroids and interferon when the body is exposed to viral infection: vitamin C (this also increases the production of lymphocytes, which cancer patients have a poor ability to make); vitamin B5 (calcium pantothenate); vitamin A, the anti-infection vitamin, which tends to shorten the duration of an illness and quite definitely increases immunity against environmental pollution; selenium – this stimulates the effectiveness of coenzyme Q10 and helps produce more antibodies; and zinc is absolutely essential to the functions of the immune system as there are over 70 enzymes in the body which are zinc-dependent, particularly for the biosynthesis of the nucleic acids RNA and DNA, it inhibits the evolution of infectious virions (viral replicas), it has a stimulating effect on all reproducing cells, and a deficiency causes a wasting away of the thymus gland.

- Nutrients and moderate sunshine to aid vitamin D synthesis.
- Nutrients to keep free radicals under control – see Chapter 17.
- Nutrients to maintain levels of antibodies: amino acids phenylalaline and tryptophan; zinc; most vitamins; pangamic acid (DMG); non-specific immune stimulants such as Pascotox; plant extracts such as echinacea, viscum, equisitum, *Vinca rosea*. An excess of cholesterol and fatty acids, or deficiencies of zinc and/or iron, can lead to a high incidence of breast cancer, prostate and colon cancers; there should therefore be a balance of saturated and unsaturated fats.
- Other nutrients will include: vitamin B6, needed for production of the nucleic acids RNA and DNA, shortage of which inhibits formation of white blood cells (T lymphocytes) and anti-body formation; and calcium, an enzyme activator – the body requires far larger quantities when there is a viral infection, and it also makes vitamin C more effective.
- You can use phytotherapy (plant and herbal extracts) to induce a high fever to increase the number of leucocytes, always under the supervision of an experienced physician.
- Lifestyle changes such as eliminating smoking and alcohol, which do a great deal of harm to the immune system.
- To aid phagocyte function take vitamin C to stimulate their motility and killing ability. It will also stimulate production of T and B cells and macrophage action. Dr Robert Cathcart in America suggests 1–3 grams daily as a maintenance dose for healthy people, but for viral diseases give up to tolerance level for a short time, then reduce to maintenance dose. For patients with advanced cancer, 10 g a day has been shown (by Drs Cameron and Pauling, 1980) to increase life expectancy fourfold, but the benefit is much reduced in patients who have had cytotoxic chemotherapy and/oir radiation treatment.

- By relaxation and/or meditation and imagery, through techniques like the Silva mind method of mind control, autosuggestion as practised by Emile Coue (see Chapter 30), or autogenic training, all of which can affect the kind and levels of hormonal secretions.

9
AUTOIMMUNE DISEASES

In autoimmune diseases the T-suppressor cells fail to do their job properly and instead of the T-killer cells reserving their efforts to attack 'foreign' substances that invade the body, for some so far unaccountable reason, they decide to attack a person's own body tissues and the cells they are supposed to protect. This is most common among people who already have an underactive immune system, and is more common in women than in men. It has also been noted that people with auto-immune diseases have a tendency to repress any negative emotions such as anger; a tendency to hide emotion also comes out strongly as a characteristic of many people who contract cancer.

THE MAJOR AUTOIMMUNE BREAKDOWN DISEASES

Rheumatoid arthritis is a disease of the whole body, not just the joints. It may be episodic, bad one day, better the next, or slowly progressive, getting gradually worse. There is a suggestion that rheumatoid arthritis is due to excess iron which allows hydroxyl free radicals to form. It is often treated with immunosuppressants, which weaken the body allowing infection or malignancies to evolve in some instances.

Systemic lupus erythematosus (SLE) is a chronic inflammatory disease in which the patient's immune system creates too many anti-bodies and, not recognising its own connective tissues or collagen, atttacks itself. Lupus erythematosus literally means red skin in the shape of a wolf, and is a description of the rash often found on both cheeks and over the bridge of the nose; the classical rash is in the shape of a butterfly. It is not a very common disease in the UK, although as diagnostic techniques are improving the apparent numbers are increasing. Symptoms sometimes come and go spontaneously, making diagnosis difficult. It mainly affects young women, and is often diag-nosed in young people who have 'growing pains' which may later turn into rheumatoid arthritis, MS or SLE. Symptoms of SLE may include:

- Rash, weakness, lack of energy, low fever, lack of appetite, frequent infections.

- Anaemias and/or low white blood cell count.
- Easy bruising as the blood's ability to clot properly is reduced.
- The heart, lungs and abdominal organs can be affected.
- Kidney disorders.
- There may possibly be convulsions and depressions, headaches and often migraines.
- Patients suffer a strong sensitivity to the sun and other forms of ultraviolet light.
- Joint symptoms occur, but are generally less severe than those in rheumatoid arthritis.

Treatment is normally by steroids, anti-malarial drugs and sometimes other immunosuppressive agents.

Diabetes mellitus is probably partly genetic and partly autoimmune in origin. In particular, type 1, juvenile-onset or insulin-dependent diabetes mellitus (IDDM) is suspected to be an autoimmune disease. In IDDM, antibodies are produced which cause destruction of beta cells responsible for producing insulin in the islets of Langherans in the pancreas. As a result, fats are burned, leading to high levels of ketones in the blood, producing acidosis. Neuropathy or nerve damage may also result. Type 2 or maturity-onset diabetes (non-insulin-dependent diabetes mellitus, NIDDM) is caused by a different mechanism and is very responsive to dietary management.

Myasthenia gravis is a progressive disease which comes under the general muscular dystrophy syndrome. It is 'almost invariably' caused by, or at least triggered off by stress, which in itself if often caused by low blood sugar levels, as well as the normal triggers of emotional or business stresses, etc. It appears to involve a defect in the production of acetylcholine, which transmits nerve impulses to the muscles; myasthenia gravis is thus a form of progressive paralysis through a defect of transmission across the gap between nerve and muscle. The symptoms include:

- Grave loss of muscle strength: first the muscles of the eyes, head, neck and mouth weaken; then those of the thorax, making breathing difficult, with possible stuttering and stammering; then weakness in other limbs, in the chewing muscles (i.e. eat first thing in the morning while muscles have some strength in them).
- The thyroid gland is sometimes enlarged, giving typical adrenal exhaustion symptoms and/or severe lack of pantothenic acid. The thyroid, if toxic, is often removed.
- The thymus gland may be enlarged (hypertrophy), instead of almost atrophying as normal in adults.

- There may be early fatigue, particularly after repetitive movements, with difficulty in keeping the upper eyelids open and mouth closed.
- There may be excessive white blood corpuscles in the blood.

Dietary suggestions include six small high-protein meals daily, including lambs' liver, egg yolks and pumpkin seeds, all of which are good sources of choline. Supplements should include vitamin B, particularly B3, vitamin E, magnesium, potassium and some manganese at each meal, and lecithin, which contains choline. For stress give vitamin C, vitamin B5 and vitamins B2 and B6. Homoeopathic curare 6-30 C in stages can also be of help.

Myalgic encephalomyelitis (ME) and the post-viral fatigue syndrome (PVFS) are covered separately in the next chapter.

Other ailments thought to come under the general heading of auto-immune diseases include Addison's disease, cystic fibrosis, Graves' disease, scleroderma (hard skin patches), aspermatogenesis (when a man produces antibodies against his own sperm, resulting in sterility), Sjögren's syndrome, some schizophrenia, some allergies and anaemias and some kidney diseases.

AIDS

Acquired immunodeficiency syndrome (AIDS) and AIDS-related conditions are diseases which present very complicated clinical pictures and generally affect the organism as a whole.

Patients with autoimmune breakdown diseases need a very positive clinical approach as many of them have battled with their illness for a long time and are emotionally and mentally drained.

10
MYALGIC ENCEPHALOMYELITIS AND POST-VIRAL FATIGUE SYNDROME

Otherwise known as Royal Free Disease (or unkindly called shirkers disease, as many doctors consider it purely a psychosomatic ailment, while others do not recognise it at all), this is a syndrome, a collection of symptoms, of which one is the post-viral fatigue syndrome. This is a long-term debilitating disorder of the central nervous system (brain and spinal cord) and there are about 100,000 people in the UK with it. The diagnosed and suspected number of cases is growing alarmingly.

VIRUSES AND DISEASE

Everyone, whether they know it or not, has between two and seven viral infections every year, with recovery occurring in most cases. There are thousands of viruses, absolutely minute beings, which produce illnesses such as measles, rubella, mumps, flu, hepatitis A and B, chickenpox, the common cold. But infection only occurs if:

- Enough virus gets into the body.
- The patient is susceptible.
- The virus is able to replicate.

Usually an attack by one virus makes that person immune to further attacks by that particular kind of virus. Unfortunately different viruses can cause similar ailments, for example there are hundreds of different viruses that cause the common cold, so having a disease once does not guarantee that you won't get it again.

Viruses can only replicate within living cells, using the cell's biochemical systems to produce the components for further viruses which are then released from the cell, allowing the whole procedure to be repeated. While the viruses are multiplying (during the incubation period of a disease) they spread to specific parts of the body which they selectively attack (e.g. the hepatitis virus attacks the liver), and doctors can assess which virus is on the attack by the symptoms produced and the organs affected.

Sometimes, however, problems continue to occur many months, or years, after the initial viral attack. By then there is no clinical sign of infection, only signs that the immune system is abnormal. PVFS can then be diagnosed through the characteristic history of the patient, with evidence of a past viral infection. There is then a prolonged period of ill health, when the symptoms are not due to the acute infection but to the effects that infection had on the body. The patient may have debilitating symptoms of excessive tiredness and poor recovery after minor exercise, which may result in twitching muscles, or pain and burning in muscles. Other symptoms which may arise might include:

- Inability to concentrate, and a poor memory.
- Dizziness when travelling in a car, leading to a feeling of disorientation.
- Depression, paranoia and contemplation of suicide.

Traditional medicine cannot normally detect such a viral infection that continues years after the initial infection, but research by Professor James Mowbray at St Mary's Hospital in London has found evidence, in over half their ME patients, of constant infection by enteroviruses, i.e. the enterovirus persists in the patient for many years.

CAUSES OF ME

The following viruses have been implicated in ME.

- Epstein-Barr virus, which causes infectious mononucleosis – usually an illness of adolescents, and often called the 'kissing disease' as infection is often passed on in saliva during a kiss – and also glandular fever, which usually occurs in childhood or adolescence.
- Coxsackie viruses, spread from the faeces of infected persons. Generally the illness lasts only a few days or weeks, but occasionally symptoms persist and PVFS develops.
- Enteroviruses. These are small viruses which live in the gut but affect other organs such as the liver, pancreas, spleen or lungs. There are about 75 different varieties. Initially they may present themselves as a respiratory tract infection (colds, flu-like illnesses, sore throat, runny nose, aches and pains, etc., coughs).

In acute-onset ME probably 20 per cent of cases at least are related to glandular fever. In slow-onset ME people may have digestive problems and/or irritable bowel syndrome but only a little fatigue, but still may go on to develop ME slowly.

Let us look at the two groups of viruses most commonly implicated in ME, the enteroviruses (which include the Coxsackie viruses) and the Epstein-Barr virus.

Enteroviruses inhabit the gastrointestinal tract and its lining, and their presence there may be encouraged if there are too many of the wrong organisms in the gut, of which the most significant are the candida species. There is evidence that candida, a type of yeast, is active on the cell lining of the gut wall, because the gut wall gets covered with a pseudowall of foreign matter, mainly made up of glutenous compounds and decayed matter from plant and animal sources. (In a biopsy of the gut wall lining, about half of the cellular weight of that lining is made up of foreign proteins.)

Enteroviruses survive storage, freezing, disinfectants, water and sewage treatments, i.e. they are very tough. People most likely to get infected with these viruses include:

- Those in contact with children (parents, teachers, welfare officers, etc.).
- Those who are living in or in contact with insanitary conditions.
- Those who cannot rest when ill, e.g. mothers of small children, teachers, students, etc.

Enteroviral diseases include:

- 'Summer' flu (headaches, sore throats, diarrhoea).
- Colds, laryngitis, bronchitis, pneumonia.
- Ear and sinus infections.
- Glandular fever.
- Meningitis, encephalitis.
- Muscle weaknesses, paralysis, Bornholm disease.
- Appendicitis, hepatitis, pancreatitis.
- Inflammation of thyroid or parotid glands, testes or ovaries.
- Arthritis.
- MS, motor neurone disease, cerebral ataxia.

They usually start in the mouth and move down into the gastrointestinal tract. A large percentage may result in upper respiratory tract infection, and some of these may then go on to develop ME.

If, however, there is much stress, these enteroviruses will spread, via the bloodstream, to target organs which may be anywhere in the body:

- In the muscles, with the result that there is a build-up of lactic acid leading to weakness, aching and incoordination. (However, many ME patients have no muscle pains.)

- In the brain many functions are interfered with, such as the regulation of heartbeat (it is not uncommon to have abnormal heart rhythms with PVFS), temperature control, respiration, blood pressure, sleep rhythm. Pain perception may be abnormal, as also may be short-term memory, concentration and emotional control.

Stress-induced enteroviral complications can result from:

- Strenuous exercise.
- Immunosuppression, through the use of steroids, anti-inflammatory drugs, anti-cancer drugs.
- Secondary infections such as measles, chickenpox, flu.
- Anaesthetics, vaccinations, surgery.

ME itself is not infectious. It is the enterovirus-induced flu which may spread in an epidemic; people whose immune system is poor catch it, and some then go on to develop ME.

Geographically, enterovirus infections are worse in cool climates than in the tropics where, due to poor sanitation causing widespread infection, most children develop a natural immunity. In cool climates infection is less prevalent but if adults do contract it they get it in a more severe form.

There is evidence, from their response to antibiotics (that kill bacteria but not viruses), that ME patients suffer from persistent bacterial infection in the gut as well as viral infections and candida. It appears that this is one of the reasons why it is so hard to ascertain what viruses are present, as it seems to depend so much on what the conditions are that they encounter in the individual as to what type of virus that person is likely to culture. Research shows that many bowel problems are associated with ME.

Infectious mononucleosis – often confused with glandular fever – is caused by the Epstein-Barr virus and often brings out symptoms that suggest it is cancer or leukaemia; in fact some doctors think it is cancer, but one that the body's immune system can control. Entry into the body is through:

- Respiratory tract, through coughs, sneezes, speaking, shaking hands of contaminated person, saliva, by sharing towels, etc.
- Alimentary tract, where the virus multiplies and passes into the faeces – which may in turn contaminate drinking water or, through discharge of untreated sewage, contaminate shellfish such as oysters; or contamination may be passed on through the hands of infected food handlers.

- The skin, e.g. via breaks in the skin caused by herpes (cold sores).
- Sharing of needles by drug addicts, and occasionally from blood transfusions.

POST-VIRAL FATIGUE SYNDROME

Many patients with post-viral fatigue syndrome (PVFS) are unjustly accused of malingering, but there is now a blood test as a result of research at St Mary's Hospital, London, which can confirm whether or not a person is suffering from PVFS. This has shown that it is not uncommon for more than one member of the family to have PVFS.

The symptoms of PVFS are as follows:

- Fatigue (asthenia), total exhaustion.
- General feeling of malaise, of feeling unwell; a 'never felt so ill' feeling.
- Excessive tiredness and exhaustion.
- Increased sweating.
- Muscle pain, weakness, tremors, twitches, heaviness, cramp, burning.
- Severe myalgia (muscular pain) in arms and legs, which gets increasingly worse, is found in 30 per cent of patients.
- Persistent feeling of unsteadiness, vertigo.
- Abnormal vascular function, i.e. cold or very warm hands and feet.
- Pallor in the face.
- Neurological symptoms such as headaches, light-headedness, dizziness, sensitivity to temperature, ringing in the ears, mental stupefaction.
- Blurred vision, sore eyes, possible difficulty in focusing due to fatigue of the ciliary muscles and other eye symptoms such as flashing lights.
- Difficulty of speaking, or finding the right words.
- Fears, depression, poor concentration, paranoia – when patients find it difficult to understand how people round them cannot understand their illness, to the point when they contemplate suicide.
- Feelings of frustration, resentment, self-anger, self-pity, alternating with feelings of resignation, apathy or optimism.
- Gastrointestinal symptoms are very common and food allergies may develop; diarrhoea, pain in the abdomen, nausea (vomiting rare).
- Cardiac and respiratory complaints such as pains in the chest, palpitations, dyspnoea.

- Headaches similar to cluster headaches.
- Loss of weight due to lack of energy to cook and/or eat.
- Other bizarre symptoms of a very individual nature, e.g. the symptoms get worse on lying down, then get worse on getting up again.
- There will be many fears, including the fear of death and cancer.

Symptoms are greatly exacerbated by stress, particularly emotional stresses. It is not fully understood how this link between stress and disease works, but it appears that a patient's emotional state may influence the function of his immune system, reducing levels of IgA antibodies and increasing the ratio of helper T cells to suppressor T cells. It is thus possible that the patient's emotional state may predispose him to a viral infection, and to prolonged recovery from that infection – some evidence has been found in patients with infectious mononucleosis.

The first step in recovery therefore involves the patient believing in himself and adopting a plan for recovery. It is necessary to accept that a person with ME or PVFS is ill, and for that person to accept that he or she is ill and that it is not all in their minds. They must accept this as a fact and that it is not necessary to 'fight it', but to accept the limitations, i.e. to rest when tired, go home, sit down, and not feel guilty about giving in. One normal symptom is to feel all right on waking up but to get progressively worse on doing any exercise.

Firstly admit that cure may take a long time – there is no hope of a quick cure, and therefore no frustration when spectacular improvement does not occur. However, eventually it is likely that full recovery will be obtained. Secondly one has to get involved with one's illness and adopt a lifestyle which will help. Any successes should be objectively recorded, to provide a boost for the future.

PVFS develops at two ages mostly, at 25–30 and 40–5. Patients are normally on the whole more active and energetic than others. Exercise, however, quickly results in exhaustion and is followed by a prolonged period during which the body recharges itself. Each person therefore has to find out the maximum exercise to undertake without causing prolonged tiredness.

Tiredness in PVFS appears to be caused by the quicker-than-usual-formation of lactic acid in muscles, which also tends to take longer to get rid of compared to normal muscles. The muscles in PVFS are thus abnormally affected and therefore normal exercise should not be undertaken, even though most people with PVFS appear to be more athetic than the average individual and look on exercise as being the way to fitness. For the first six months there should be no strenuous exercise, and lots of rest.

Sleep is vitally important. Through sleep the body is able to increase the rate of repair of damaged tissues, and there is a reduced breakdown of muscle cells. Trying to stop going to sleep is only delaying the repair processes.

Food allergies develop in patients with PVFS and can result in symptoms in almost any system in the body, e.g.:

- Sweating unrelated to exercise; fatigue that is not helped by rest.
- Swelling of various parts of the body; changes in body weight.
- Wheezing; difficulty in breathing; pains; palpitations.
- Abdominal pain; feeling full all the time or after food.
- Burning bladder, frequent urination; diarrhoea.
- Muscular aches, pains and burning (although it is quite common for ME patients not to have muscle pains).
- Joint pains, difficulty moving.
- Itchy rashes.
- Dizziness, headache, migraine, nasal catarrh, sinus problems.
- Depression, panic attacks, paranoia.

All these are similar to true PVFS symptoms, but must be distinguished from them. One way is to test for food allergies with a seven-day fast; if there is no improvement at the end of that time, then challenge with the offending foods.

People with PVFS are usually profoundly tired and exhausted after even a moderate amount of alcohol. It is thought that this may result from dilatation of the blood vessels, resulting in the pooling of blood in the muscle tissues causing a reduced oxygen supply and a build-up of harmful metabolites. PVFS sufferers cannot recover from this as quickly as people with normal muscle function. It is useful to keep a diary of the type of alcohol drunk and its effects, as some forms are tolerated better than others.

Self-help groups are useful, providing mutual help and support and a recognition that one is sick and not malingering. Members discuss ways of overcoming some of the stresses of PVFS that have been found helpful to them, and everyone's knowledge of the ailment increases.

If a patient wants to remain employed he or she must:

- Stop unnecessary exertion.
- Minimise all walking, and always walk slowly.
- Think before carrying out any physical activity, which requires a lot of energy.
- Rest or sleep at home, generally stopping all social engagements.

The ME Association suggest the following supplements are helpful towards recovery:

- Multimineral and vitamin supplement.
- Magnesium.
- Chelated zinc.
- Phosphate.
- Tryptophan to help sleep.
- Evening primrose oil.
- Acidophilus (see anti-candida treatment in Chapter 14).

Experience suggests that three-quarters of all ME patients will recover providing they strictly follow an anti-candida programme (see page 75). Using nystatin or Capricin alone will not overcome candidiasis without adhering to an anti-candida diet.

And finally, a few unrelated points:

- Constant expectation of recovery 'next week' can have a demoralising effect on both doctor and patient. Patients must recognise they are ill, and ill people need rest and patience.
- The necessary rest will give the patient more time for self-understanding.
- If the viral infection that the patient may have had originally is known, then possibly a homoeopathic nosode of that viral infection may help.
- There may be nutrient deficiencies such as zinc, magnesium, and B vitamins.
- There will almost certainly be candida infection, requiring anti-candida treatment.
- PVFS is sometimes erroneously thought to be multiple sclerosis. However in PVFS, unlike MS, it has been found that weak muscles burn up energy much faster than normal, and this would explain why people with PVFS become tired so easily and need so much rest to overcome their muscular problems.
- The great majority of ME patients eventually recover. In a study by Dr David Smith, medical adviser to the ME Association, 22 per cent recovered within two years, 39 per cent in four years, 20 per cent in six and only 14 per cent were still affected after six years.

USEFUL ADDRESSES

- The Myalgic Encephalomyelitis Association, PO Box 8, Stanford-le-Hope, Essex SS17 8EX. Amongst other activities it publishes its *ME Association Newsletter*.

II
MULTIPLE SCLEROSIS

Multiple sclerosis (MS) is a multi-factorial autoimmune disease where the defence system attacks the body it is meant to be protecting. Specifically, the myelin sheath round some of the nerves deteriorates. Sometimes it reforms spontaneously for no known reason but, if not, the body's natural response is to try and repair the damage by filling the damaged area with connective tissue (scars or sclerosis) which cannot conduct nerve impulses.

The second cranial nerve is often affected, i.e. the nerve behind the eye, giving optic or retrobulbar disease. This gives blurred vision in one eye. Sometimes remission allows perfect sight again.

The disease can affect the spinal cord in the pyramidal tract, i.e. in the bundle of nerves conveying the brain's initiation and control of movement of muscles, particularly those in the legs. This may cause a rapid onset of sudden weakness in the legs or it may increase for a week or two, remain unchanged for a few weeks, then there may be a remission period and temporary recovery. It may also result in numbness of the feet, the numbness ascending in a few days to the waist. Or it may cause a 'loss of knowledge of where a limb is'.

There may be an inability to urinate, or incontinence even when the bladder is not full, due to damage to the neural pathways in the lower part of the spine, or it may lead to impotence in men.

MS can cause disease in the brain stem, which may result in unpleasant and persistent vertigo, or disease in the cerebellum, that part of the brain which regulates movement. The latter results in loss of control of movement which becomes incoordinated, although there is no loss of strength or sensation, e.g. unsteady walking, clumsiness of hands.

GENERAL SYMPTOMS OF MS

- Pins and needles in left foot and leg.
- Weakness in knees.

- Blurring of vision of right eye.
- Balance becomes poor; tendency to stagger; lack of coordination.
- Dizzy when closing eyes.
- Itching of face.
- Lapses of memory.
- Speech difficulties.
- Bowel and bladder disorders and loss of control.
- Patient generally feels well, but tired.

Onset may be very rapid, there may be facial neuralgia (of the trigeminal nerve) on one side of the face, with brief paroxysms of great pain, 10–15 seconds at a time. There may be intense itching paroxysms of small isolated areas of skin. Hot baths or exertion may cause temporary weakness or blindness. Often the disease lasts many years, with only occasional attacks of weakness. The disease strikes young adults mainly, between 17 and 30; it is rare before 15 or after 50.

SOME POSSIBLE CAUSES OF MS

- It is often triggered by traumatic stress.
- It is possibly a result of an excess of lead or mercury in the body, although toxic metal poisoning can produce symptoms which will mimic MS; always check any suspected MS for toxic metal poisoning.
- It is possibly a result of candida overgrowth.
- It is possibly a rickettsiae infection.
- It is possibly a gluten allergy.

A deficiency of vitamin B12 may cause pernicious anaemia (diagnosable from the vitamin level in blood) with spinal cord damage, and is sometimes confused with MS. A benign tumour of the spinal cord which causes compression also looks like MS while some patients with ME are also sometimes wrongly diagnosed as having MS. (A simple test is to stand up, put your feet apart, shut your eyes and bring your feet together. If this is not possible, then it is probably MS.)

ESSENTIAL FATTY ACIDS AND MS

In MS any essential fatty acids ingested are not broken down in the correct chain of reactions that normally lead to the production of prostaglandins.

Prostaglandins, as produced normally, regulate every cell and hormone in the body and are important for the regulation of platelet production. They also help the immune system, which is compromised in MS patients. The production of prostaglandins happens in four stages, starting off with linoleic acid which is converted to gammer linolenic acid (GLA), but there are blocking agents which stop this from happening (apart from a lack of zinc). To overcome this it is necessary to go straight to the GLA stage by having a supplement such as evening primrose oil (or spirulina).

Gamma linolenic acid (GLA) is capable of altering abnormal cell membranes, including myelin sheaths, and can return them to a normal condition within a year. It is therefore important for people with MS to have GLA supplements (such as evening primrose oil) as they are inefficient at converting linoleic acid to GLA (possibly also through lack of zinc, which helps this first step in the chain).

To help the conversion of GLA into an intermediary which can lead to the production of prostaglandins, one needs:

- Vitamins B1, B2, B5, B6 (in the early stages), B12.
- Vitamin B3 to help the conversion further.
- Vitamin E, essential to prevent oxidation of unsaturated fatty acids into dangerous peroxides, which may cause demyelination.
- Vitamin C as an antioxidant, and also to help the conversion.
- Zinc, which is essential in many metabolic functions.
- Lecithin to help myelin sheath and nerve transmission.
- The amino acid carnitine, which improves fat metabolism.
- Cobalt, magnesium, manganese, iron and calcium may also be needed.
- Octacosanol, an amino acid, appears to slow down, or reverse, the disappearance of myelin sheaths (which would then 'short-circuit' the exposed nerves, leading to pain) in conditions like muscular dystrophy, myasthenia gravis and MS.
- Histidine, another amino acid, is necessary for the maintenance of myelin sheaths.
- Linusit gold for linoleic acid and fibre.

As there may be spontaneous remissions for a time, any assistance that can be given towards removing allergies, candida, deficiencies, etc. will help to lengthen these periods of remission.

DIET AND MS

- Little or no saturated fats, or animal fats.
- No dairy products except low-fat yoghourt, goats' or sheeps' milk or cheeses.

- No refined carbohydrates (e.g. white bread, cakes, biscuits, etc.).
- No sugar.
- Oils to provide the necessary linoleic acid. A daily intake of three to four tablespoons may be necessary; part may be taken as supplements and part as oil, which can be used in salad dressings, for cooking and shallow frying or roasting.
- As MS patients sometimes have an allergy to gluten it may be worth having gluten-free bread and keeping off other gluten products. This will also fit in with any anti-candida measures taken.
- Eat fish at least three times a week.
- Eat dark green vegetables, legumes, pulses (preferably raw), and salads daily.
- Eat nuts, seeds and seed oils, particularly linseed oil.
- Only a little lean meat, lambs' liver and other offal which provide a rich source of arachidonic acid should be included in the diet, provided one is not allergic to them.
- Only take alcohol in moderation, provided one is not allergic to it. (No fermented drinks.)
- No smoking, which nullifies the good effect of a diet high in essential fatty acids.

HOMOEOPATHIC REMEDIES AND MS

- Always use the constitutional remedy if known; then the following should be considered: agaricus, alumen, arg. nit., aurum met., baryta mur., causticum, curare, medorrhinum, nat. mur. (which prolongs periods of remission), phosphorus, plumbum, sulphur.
- Kali bich. is useful for detoxifying microbial toxins affecting the nervous system during progressive muscular atrophy.
- As there may be a connection between the onset of MS and an attack of measles, morbillinum might also be useful where measles preceded the onset of muscular weakness.
- For suppressed immune system use nux. vom. in the morning and sulphur in the evening.

EXERCISE AND MS

One of the primary symptoms of MS, as outlined earlier in this chapter, is that the patient feels well but tired.

For muscles to work, they need oxygen, which they obtain from glucose. This glucose is transported to the muscles in the bloodstream, which flows more readily as a result of exercise. Paradoxically, therefore, some exercise is beneficial in overcoming fatigue, preferably with some rest periods in between. The best thing is to exercise gently; do not over-exercise to the point of fatigue.

Remember, a muscle unused is a muscle we lose.

OTHER REMEDIES

Dr Arthur Kaslow of Solvang, California, employs a modified kind of acupuncture. A modestly charged probe-like instrument is used on 'response' points just off the classical acupuncture meridians. Each person has individual response points, but, once they have been found and energised, movement is returned to parts of the body that had become unusable or weak. A patient can carry out a programme on himself at home with a stimulator. This means that there is not a final and permanent destruction of part of the nervous system at all, at least in the early stages.

Dr Kaslow also found that there was a strong connection between MS and food allergies; even that eating large amounts of a food to which one is normally tolerant could trigger off symptoms. The result was a fairly rapid relapse or show of symptoms. He suggested the 'eight mini-food programme' in which a person can eat from two teaspoons to two tablespoons of eight different foods, i.e. it is a quantity as well as a quality problem, and most people can eat, *in small amounts*, foods of which they were formerly intolerant. Certain foods he found were bad, i.e. red meat, bread, sugar and sweets. (The body needs B-complex vitamins to metabolise sugar and it is thought that these vitamins are drawn out of the myelin tissues. As there is a deterioration of the insulation round the nerves (the myelin sheath) in MS, such withdrawal will only make matters worse. MS patients may therefore be deficient in B vitamins.)

Dr Maurice Mandell, clinical ecologist, has been able to induce, in minutes or hours, flare-ups of patients' normal symptoms of MS by exposing them to various allergens. As a corollary, allergic desensitisation to airborne allergens have proved helpful for MS sufferers, together with desensitisation to chemicals and some dietary intakes.

Dr Carton Fredericks suggests that in early cases of MS, a diet high in oily fish, e.g. mackerel, trout, salmon, sardines, is helpful. In MS there is a 'sludging' of blood, impairing circulation in a similar manner to thrombosis (blood clotting) and the eicosapentaenoic acid in fish oil is a factor which reduces the tendency towards excessive adhesion of blood platelets.

If the small intestine is overgrown with enteroviruses, bacteria and fungi, it is possible for residues of these organisms to leak byproducts into the bloodstream and eventually for toxic deposits of this material to lodge along the nerve pathways. Infiltration of this fibrous, acidic and toxic material can then form fibrositis or fibroids.

This fibrous tissue however is not inert, but often carries the residue of genetic material, plus the proteins of long-dead colonies of bacteria and fungi which still contain mycotoxins (toxic compounds from yeasts and fungi), and it is these secretions which make inroads into the nervous system. Furthermore, we now know that people with MS always have a high level of yeast growth in the body, so if they can control and regulate the amount of yeast growth in the body, they can control many of the symptoms. Yeast colonies in fact are short-lived, so if you can repeatedly interrupt the life-cycle, and continue with anti-fungal policy, there comes a point where they do not overgrow again. The nerve sheath can then carry the energy messages and fibrillate, loosening the fibrous material that has built up around them so that that nerve passage becomes free again and able to regulate and send the desired commands. It is marvellous to witness the changes which are clearly the product of more adequate nerve-pathway opening. A gluten-free diet, plus a lot of polyunsaturated fats and some saturated ones – coconut oil, unsalted butter, olive oil, sesame oil, linseed oil (i.e. all those that do not oxidise easily) – will help.

At Surrey University samples from MS patients have been analysed, showing a significant shortage of zinc, copper, cobalt and magnesium. Through a dietary programme you can institute changes which will increase the absorption of the good nutrients and decrease the appearance of the harmful intestinal flora. Replenishing the good gut flora in this way can directly help the myelin sheathing to repair and often stops the destructive process seen in MS.

USEFUL ADDRESSES

- ARMS (Action for Research into MS), 71 Gray's Inn Road, London WC1X 8TR.
- ARMS telephone counselling service, 071-586 2255.
- Action for ARMS Research, Dartmouth Street, London SW1, 071-222 3224.
- The MS Society of Great Britain, 286 Munster Road, London SW6 6AP, 071-381 4022.

12
SCHIZOPHRENIA

Schizophrenia is a common and disabling ailment, affecting one in 100 people in the UK, often isolating people from those around them and making it very difficult for sufferers to hold down a job, marry, raise a family or live independently. Some people do recover, but generally schizophrenics have a series of attacks and remain ill to some extent throughout their lives.

SYMPTOMS OF SCHIZOPHRENIA

Schizophrenia is not a question of having a 'split personality', as the popular image would have it. Instead, the sufferer may:

- Hear voices that no one else can hear.
- Think that objects, events or people control their thoughts or actions, in a way that cannot be explained.
- Think in a confused and muddled manner. Speech may be hard to follow.
- Have an inability to have or to show feelings, or have feelings which are out of place.
- Hide away from people.
- Be afflicted with a loss of energy, self-neglect.

Physical symptoms include:

- Loss of ability to dream or remember dreams after waking.
- Abdominal pain in left upper side of abdomen.
- Constipation.
- Inability to tan in sunlight; itching in sunlight.
- Malformation of knee cartilages.
- Joint pains; tremors, muscle spasms.
- May be impotent.
- White spots on fingernails.
- Anaemia, in which vitamin B6 and not iron is necessary.
- Some have eyes which follow movements not smoothly but with a jagged pattern.

Note that a high proportion of schizophrenics are left-handed.

Diagnosis of schizophrenia will take into account the following:

- Feeling of being overwhelmingly tired in the day and over-active at night. Excessive tiredness for no apparent reason is an early symptom, although unfortunately this is also a symptom of a number of degenerative diseases and of candida infection.
- Chronic illness lasting at least six months.
- Irritability over trivial matters, especially towards members of the family; undue suspicion of people, i.e. paranoid feelings.
- Presence of delusions, hallucinations, frightening thoughts or incomprehensible speech.
- A history of poor work and poor concentration.
- A feeling of often being anxious, panicky, depressed, weepy or suicidal.
- Onset usually before 40 years of age.

CAUSES OF SCHIZOPHRENIA

Causes may include:

- A severe imbalance of metals and minerals in the body, particularly a shortage of zinc required to balance excess of copper.
- Low blood sugar.
- Shortage of vitamin B6 and C.
- Possibly a biochemically induced disease similar in symptoms to pellagra (curable by vitamin B3).
- Lithium imbalance and vanadium toxicity which are often reported in the literature.

Furthermore, it may:

- Sometimes be inherited.
- Be an allergy to gluten, similar to coeliac disease.
- Be due to altered intestinal permeability, thereby allowing partially digested food to find its way into the blood circulation and thence into the brain. This may be due to candida infection in the gut; many of the symptoms of candida infection are similar to those of schizophrenia.
- Possibly be a deficiency in prostaglandin E1.
- Result from a weakening of the immune system; schizophrenics are often physically ill, showing that their body as a whole, as well as their brain, is affected.

Schizophrenia is triggered off sometimes by stressful events, good or bad, and by many other events which bring on schizophrenia in people who have a predisposition to it. It seems to run in families. Strong evidence is emerging that it may be a genetically transmitted disease or the result of birth trauma (e.g. winter births). There may possibly be an excess of brain dopamine (a precursor of adrenaline) production as a trigger factor.

TREATMENT FOR SCHIZOPHRENIA

Treatment, apart from neuroleptic drugs, includes:

- Gluten-free and milk-free diet may be beneficial. (Note there may be powdered milk in so-called 'gluten-free' flours.)
- Evening primrose oil, e.g. Efamol.
- Vitamin C.
- Vitamin B6.
- Vitamin B3 potentiates (increases the effects of) drugs, so less tranquillisers are required, with a reduction in side effects.
- Zinc.
- The amino acid cystine has had good results and helped paranoia and hallucinations.
- Homoeopathic remedies include agaricus, *Cannabis indica*, anacardium; possibly hyoscyamus, nat. sulph.
- Bach flower remedies: 26, rock rose for terror: 2, aspen for fear of unknown terrors; 15, holly, for suspicion, revenge, vexation.

USEFUL ADDRESSES

- National Schizophrenia Fellowship, 78 Victoria Road, Surbiton, Surrey KT6 4NS, is a charity devoted to supporting carers, relatives and sufferers of schizophrenia. Information and advice are available.
- SANE (Schizophrenia: A National Emergency), 5th Floor, 120 Regent Street, London W1A 5FE, is a charity formed to raise public awareness of problems with schizophrenia, to promote care for victims and their families, and to help research towards a cure.
- Schizophrenia Association of Great Britain, International Schizophrenia Centre, Hydryd, The Crescent, Bangor, Gwynnedd LL75 2AG, Wales.

13
MOTOR NEURONE DISEASE

Motor neurone disease is a degenerative disease and there is no known effective treatment, although there are measures that can help. It is a form of paralysis, possibly caused by some virus infection, which generally attacks people in middle life. The disease may at some time spontaneously halt its degenerative process, for some as yet unknown reason. This does give a measure of hope.

It is a degeneration of the grey matter of the spinal cord and brain, and therefore of the corresponding peripheral motor nerves which carry messages from the central nervous system to the muscles, resulting in the wasting of those muscles which are operated by these nerves. There may be a twitching of some muscles around the shoulder. It is virtually the same as progressive muscular atrophy, which starts as a wasting of the hand muscles and may take some years before it spreads to other parts of the body; sometimes, though, it is rapid and widespread, finally affecting the muscles of the neck and throat, making it increasingly difficult to speak or swallow correctly so that some food may go down the wrong way, ending up in the lungs. (To help counteract this choking avoid very hot or sweet foods, avoid salt and always have a cup of water handy.) Bulbar paralysis is similar.

REMEDIES FOR MOTOR NEURONE DISEASE

Exercise as much as possible, and massage muscles. For the pain take:

- Vitamin C, particularly for easing pain in brain tissues.
- Homoeopathic hypericum, arnica and vanadium may well be helpful.
- Vitamin B (non-yeast) complex.
- The trace elements copper, magnesium, zinc, cobalt, selenium, molybdenum have all been found to be lacking in people with motor neurone disease and appropriate supplementation with them will also probably be helpful.

The extreme shortages of trace elements in people with this disease suggest that there is a faulty absorption mechanism. The gut is often contaminated by enteroviruses, bacteria and fungi, which cannot absorb the fine nutrients that are needed for nerve and grey matter repair; they get leached out of the body, while all the coarser material consisting of undigested food and breakdown products, foreign proteins, bacteria, fungi and viruses gets into the blood. Furthermore, enteroviruses and remnants of fungi and bacteroides can attack the neural system, leading to neurological disease. (See Chapter 14 on measures to counteract candida infestation and fungal toxaemia.)

USEFUL ADDRESSES

The Motor Neurone Disease Association, 61 Derngate, Northampton NN1 1UE, can help with advice.

14
CANDIDA

If you suffer from undiagnosed medical symptoms such as depression, headaches without any apparent reason, hayfever, sore throats, tightness in the chest, vaginal burning, forgetfulness, bloating of the stomach, chronic diarrhoea or constipation, asthma, inability to cope, lethargy, or menstrual problems, then the probability is that you are one of the 25 per cent of the population who have an overgrowth of *Candida albicans* in their systems. Other conditions that suggest candidiasis are poor coordination, spots in front of the eyes, recurring ear infection, muscle aches, swelling in the joints, bad breath, indigestion, allergic reactions to foods, chemicals and inhalants. It is thus a factor behind a surprising number of ailments. Indeed polysystemic chronic candidiasis (PCC) is nowadays a common occurrence amongst people whose immune systems have broken down.

WHAT EXACTLY IS CANDIDA?

Candida albicans is a natural yeast/fungus which should constitute 10–15 per cent of the normal intestinal flora. A balance is maintained by the friendly bacteria in the intestinal tract, which keep candida in check by competing for food. It lives on and in humans, and relies on using oxygen to help it 'burn' its 'fuel' – in this case the human mucous membranes.

It is a dimorphic organism. In the yeast form there is no root formation, but in its fungal form it produces rhizoids similar to roots which can penetrate the mucosa of the tissues of the intestines or any other organ that is invaded.

Candida is a mould that is everywhere. If it is given living conditions in the human body, and the type of food it likes and sufficient room to grow, it will proliferate greatly and swamp the more beneficial bacteria we rely on for our health and well being. This may then lead in the short term to oral thrush or vaginitis, but if the overgrowth is sustained it will lead to PCC.

The candida fungus ordinarily grows as a yeast-like form, but under conditions of overgrowth it grows fibres (mycelia) which embed themselves in the walls of the intestines, particularly in the first part of the intestines, i.e. the duodenum and jejunum. These mycelia punch holes through which waste products excreted by bacteria pass into the blood. These substances are very carcinogenic, and are some of the most pernicious substances known to man. Cancer will not appear unless pathogenic infection is extensive in the small intestines, and this applies wherever the cancer may be. Many other problems, such as pain and bloating, disappear when treated with anti-fungal substances.

Toxins excreted by the candida fungus puncture the body cells, which change their shape and begin to oxidise (for example if you cut an apple or a vegetable it begins to grow brown; this is oxidation), giving rise to inflammation (anything with an 'itis', such as laryngitis, tonsilitis, bronchitis, otitis, etc.), showing that the body is trying to get rid of these oxidising cells. The cells can get very distorted in the process and toxins pierce the cell walls and penetrate right into the genetic package. The cells then burst and tiny bits of genetic information ooze out or, when toxins are intensely active, the cells are split in half and the genetic package is then opened, accelerating cell division. The natural inclination of genes is to live and be part of a cell, so they gather plasma material around them in order to try and form a new cell, but the result is an incomplete process that has not the necessary genetic information to reproduce itself correctly, in accord with a particular type of chromosome memory.

There are about 200 different species of 'good' or beneficial bacteria in the gut (the intestines). Their task is to help in the breakdown, processing and transport of nutrients, augmenting the work of the digestive enzymes. Once the nutrients are in a form which the body can deal with they are then absorbed across the gut wall into the bloodstream and lymphatic system, this process being aided by the villi of the gut wall. These villi are finger-like or hair-like projections of the wall into the cavity of the gut, and there are millions of them, the overall effect being to increase the surface area for absorption by an enormous factor.

However, if an overgrowth of pathogens, especially the candida species, is allowed to build up in the gut it can form sticky deposits, consisting of candida, dead bacteria, waste products of other microorganisms, mucus, gluten, attached to the intestinal wall. These deposits gradually build up until eventually a solid shell is formed on the absorptive lining of the intestines, which effectively and severely limits the range and amount of nutrients the gut wall can absorb.

This means that however good one's diet is, one is not going to get the nutrients from it, the small intestines (in particular the section containing the collection of small glands called Peyer's patches) being the part of the body where nutrients can be, and are in a form to be, absorbed into the blood, which then carries them to all the cells of the body. As the villi cannot now do their job, the result is that the nutrients in food will not get through to the bloodstream. This happens particularly in cancer patients and other degenerative diseases.

WHAT IS CANDIDA'S JOB?

The prime object of all bacteria in the gut is to assist in the breakdown of food into amino acids, vitamins and minerals, sugars and fatty acids so that these biochemical building blocks can be transported from our gut into the blood. If we allow bad bacteria to colonise the gut our digestion of food is compromised so that larger molecules – starches, sugars, proteins and fats, bound up with calcium and toxins such as the chemicals in our food – pass into our bloodstream. These larger chemical units or bonds can then act as toxins within the body, for example getting into the brain via the blood/brain barrier in the case of PVFS, MND, ALD, etc.

Each type of bacteria in the gut thrives on a specific type of food. If therefore a person keeps eating the type of foods that feed the wrong bacteria, then that particular organism will thrive.

Everyone has a certain amount of candida, about 10 to 15 per cent of the total intestinal bacterial flora, in their systems. (There are about 3½ lb of bacteria in the intestines altogether.) Candida's specific job is the processing of sugars, starches and mucoproteins. However, candida is an opportunistic organism, so if something occurs to upset the delicate intestinal balance it will quickly gain a firmer foothold in the body, colonising the gastrointestinal and genitourinary tracts, as well as, very commonly, the mouth and throat. It can also invade other organs, which it colonises insidiously.

In medical school, students used to be taught that it was only a minor problem in the genital area and the intestinal tract. It was thought to be primarily a problem with women, but men, too, can develop it, as well as children who, after treatment with antibiotics, can develop a white coating on the tongue. These complaints are referred to as thrush. Candida can also co-exist alongside other diseases, such as herpes, eczema and athlete's foot.

A person with advanced cancer may have up to 100 per cent *Candida albicans* or *tropicalis* and other such parasitic organisms in the gut, therefore leaving no room for other beneficial bacteria. Indeed, one hypothesis is that degenerative diseases such as MS, rheumatoid arthritis, schizophrenia, mucopolysaccharide disease, cerebral palsy and cancer develop as a result of toxins passing into the blood through the metabolic activity of fungi, bacteria and enteroviruses as principal precursors for disease to evolve.

POLYSYSTEMIC CHRONIC CANDIDIASIS

The existence of polysystemic chronic candidiasis (PCC) as a disease itself has only just begun to be recognised. The mechanism whereby the major organ systems of the body appear to become invaded by candida is not fully understood, but the damage it causes is severe. One of the reasons behind the lack of recognition of candida species as a cause of so much ill health is precisely because they are ordinarily found in the intestines anyway. The mere presence of candida is not therefore a cause for alarm, as it is normally kept in balance by the 'friendly' bacteria such as acidophilus or bifidobacteria. As explained above, it has long been recognised as the cause of local ailments, such as oral thrush in babies and vaginal thrush in women, but it has not before been acknowledged to cause general symptoms of many different kinds.

If candida is not treated it will continue to grow. It will not get better if it is left unchecked. There are well-documented cases showing it is capable of producing alcohol and chemical derivatives, keeping its victims virtually drunk and mentally confused for years. Many people thought to be mentally ill are now found to be suffering from acute PCC problems.

Contamination by candida in fact starts very early in life, even in the formative months in the womb, so that by the time the child is born there are symptoms that indicate there is a problem. Very often medical diagnosis and treatment is difficult and it is not dealt with, except perhaps with antibiotics or nystatin, but these measures are not much use if they are not followed up with the correct nutrition – and in any case, broad spectrum antibiotics only kill off the bacteria and allow more candida growth. Candida can in fact be found on any mucous membrane, both internally, particularly in the digestive tract, and externally in any body openings and on the skin. Its best known form is recognised as oral or vaginal (otherwise called candidiasis or moniliasis) infections.

The key to the candida problem is that it congests the bowels and produces toxins which remain in the blood for some considerable time, and do not concentrate anywhere in particular. If, however, someone has a fungal infection in internal organs and/or systems, it may be an indication that the toxins have been transported and succeeded in creating 'pools' of toxic waste in different parts of the body. It may look on a scan like a tumour, but actually it forms 'nests' of microorganisms, nestling and feeding inside a case of fibrous matted, fungal exudations from successive colonies that have died back. Under such circumstances the increasing load of toxins caused by an overgrowth of candida puts a strain on the lymph nodes, where the body is trying to filter out toxins of all kinds. These nodes are often therefore the main centres where cysts or tumours start.

Candida flourishes and changes to a dangerous fungal form in both over-acid and over-alkaline conditions, but the character of fungal secretions under each condition will be different. In an over-acid person the secretions will be chemically looser, while in an over-alkaline system all the residues of the metabolism will become very sticky and adhere to the contours of whatever body system has become weakened. There will then follow a hardening, toughening process, probably with fibroid formation.

The toxic effects of candida include the manufacture of acetaldehyde, and other poisons which can produce both clear clinical and analytical profiles of candida infection (the homoeopathic nosode of acetaldehyde should be useful here – see page 246).

WHAT CAUSES CANDIDA TO PROLIFERATE?

- Any weakening of the immune system, for example as a result of:
    Radiation or chemotherapy treatment for cancer, surgery, catheter feeding.
    Steroids (which are synthetic hormones) such as cortisone or anabolic steroids in food or medication, and especially in the contraceptive pill.
    Antibiotics given as personal medication or to animals whose meat is eaten. These destroy beneficial bacteria as well as disease organisms.
    Underlying inherited or acquired deficiency in the immune system, or depletion of the immune system through continued onslaught by the candida.
- During any periods of stress people are more open to infection, and then it has been found that candida increases.
- Where there is any excess of sugar in the blood, such as is found in diabetics.
- Regular use of the contraceptive pill.
- Changes in the acidity of the stomach, due to convenience foods which may make the stomach either too acid or too alkaline.
- Poor nutrition, whereby the body is flooded with an excess of carbo-

hydrates, on which candida thrives, or a diet of foods containing yeasts and moulds, or through taking excess alcohol or drugs.
- Living in damp mouldy houses where fungi and mould spores can trigger candida overgrowth.
- In infancy the immune system is immature and a baby may become 'inoculated' with candida during birth if the mother's genital areas are infected.
- During pregnancy.
- In old age the immune system may not be 100 per cent effective.
- Deficiency of immunoglobulin A (an important antibody).
- Pesticide-laden tap water, or tap water with high levels of chlorine.
- General run-down condition.
- Insufficient gastric acid in the stomach.

SYMPTOMS WHICH MAY INDICATE CHRONIC CANDIDIASIS
- Fatigue, lethargy, irritability, headaches, migraines.
- Joint pains, with or without swelling; muscle pains.
- Nettle rash and hives.
- Irritable bowel syndrome.
- Upper abdominal discomfort or burning.
- Worsening of symptoms after eating refined carbohydrates and heavily yeasted foods.
- Sensitivity to chemicals, e.g. petrol fumes, paint, cigarette smoke, etc.
- Craving for refined carbohydrates and/or alcohol; alcohol intolerance.
- A history of oral thrush.
- Recurrent vaginal thrush/vulvar itching; anal itching.
- Recurrent cystitis, with negative bacterial cultures.
- Fungal nail or skin infections such as athlete's foot, etc.
- Iron or zinc deficiency.
- Onset of problems during, or shortly after, pregnancy.
- Sexual partner has candida problems.
- Symptoms precipitated by antibiotics; a history of excessive, repeated or long-term use of antibiotics.
- Symptoms worse in low or damp places, or near new-mown lawns, raked-up leaves or on days when the atmosphere is damp and dank (which are all symptoms of mould allergy).

Other symptoms implying there is probably candida infection include:

- Adult-onset allergies.
- Persistent drowsiness.
- Mood swings.
- Belching and wind.
- Bad breath, dry mouth and/or throat.
- Total inability to concentrate.
- 'Out of body' experiences; 'spacey' feelings.
- Alternating feverish activity or inaction.
- Longstanding adult acne; joint pains; recurrent migraines, etc.

For those who diagnose from the iris, candida infection may show up as a dark heterochromic stomach area. There may be an intense white line to the autonomic nerve wreath; there may be flares from the wreath and yellowish discolourations.

Candida may be a major factor in:

- Acne, white spots and coating on tongue; athlete's foot.
- Female problems such as vaginitis, thrush (oral and vaginal), endometriosis, cystitis; inflammation of the womb, Fallopian tubes or ovaries.
- Menstrual bleeding and cramps.
- Bowel symptoms, e.g. bloating, diarrhoea and/or constipation, abdominal noises, indigestion and acid stomach, 'spastic colon'.
- Headaches, fatigue, poor memory.
- Mental symptoms such as depression, irritability, 'neurotic' outlook.
- Allergies.
- Numbness; tingling in muscles.
- Recurrent sore throat and nasal congestion.
- Unaccountable aches and swellings in joints.
- ME; almost invariably there is mould sensitivity in ME patients, as well as severe infections.

It appears that many forms of ill health will not proliferate unless candida infection is present in the mucous membranes, particularly in the small intestines. This applies wherever the illness may be.

Candida is always present systemically in people with allergies, ME, or any malignant disease. Candida is, incidentally, very prevalent in leukaemia and AIDS patients and is found in most children with chronic complaints.

TREATMENT OF CANDIDA INFECTIONS

Always take a multiple culture of beneficial symbiotic bacteria such as Lactobacillus acidophilus and bifido (2 grams a day between meals as a supplement) or in Piima yoghourt, following the use of broad spectrum antibiotics (for a period of at least six weeks), following radiation therapy or chemotherapy (during which candida proliferates considerably), and following any gastroenteritis or diarrhoea.

Acidophilus thermophilus, bulgaricus and bifido bacteria normally exist in the intestines, where they are extremely beneficial, but poor diet, antibiotics and strong drugs can disturb the balance of the bacteria and allow pathogenic organisms to take over, resulting in lower vitality associated with low levels of the 'good' bacteria.

The acidophilus supplements (or Piima yoghourt) is required to increase the supply of healthy bacteria (*Lactobacillus acidophilus* and/or bifidobacteria) which will:

- Make the intestines more efficient at their job of sorting out nutrients required by the body.
- Produce natural antibiotics which inhibit many known pathogens.
- Help reduce cholesterol levels.
- Detoxify unhealthy material in the diet.
- Produce enzymes to help in the digestion of food and breakdown of lactose – it will therefore help people with an intolerance to lactose.
- Produce B vitamins.
- Help to neutralise toxic environmental factors.

Anyone who has been diagnosed as having candida overgrowth should, even after appropriate treatment, keep up the daily use of protective cultures to maintain a correct balance of healthy flora, because quantities of bacteria, both healthy and pathogenic (disease producing) are excreted daily. Piima yoghourt supplies all necessary 'good' bacteria (see notes on Piima on page 242).

Always make sure you have a yeast-free diet. Brewers yeast should not be taken by anyone suffering from candida.

Take biotin and/or the natural fatty acid oleic acid, as in olive oil; lack of the latter may cause the yeast form of candida to change to the fungal form. Biotin forces candida cells to adopt a compact round shape; it is only when they become filamentous do they render the intestines leaky and capable of absorbing only partially digested food and waste matter. A deficiency of biotin may show up as dermatitis of a greyish dry flaky appearance.

Aloe vera can be taken to reduce yeast organisms (a dessertspoonful in water twice daily). It also appears to reduce any inflammations, and has natural healing powers. It contains naturally bound germanium in it.

Nystatin is a powerful killer of yeast, but in doing so the dead yeasts release toxins which may cause unpleasant side effects. Also it does not replace candida with beneficial flora, so acidophilus and/or bifidobacteria supplements are still required or else the candida will return. Treatment with nystatin should continue for at least eight weeks, when noticeable improvement should be seen; it should be taken between meals or at least one hour before meals.

Quite often nystatin may be under-dosed; the minimum dose should be half a teaspoonful four times daily. Symptoms of underdosing will include tiredness, headaches, lethargy, depression, generalised aches and pains. Tablets are of little use; always take nystatin in powder form or, better still, have it injected. As nystatin appears to inactivate the B vitamins, do not take them at the same time of day. It is probably best to stay on nystatin for three months or more, having periods of a week or two on and then off for a week before taking it again. It is useful to start an anti-candida diet at least two weeks before starting treatment with nystatin, in order to minimise the natural reactions following the treatment.

Nystatin is only available in the UK on prescription at the time of writing. It has been found that some strains of candida have already become resistant to nystatin.

Caprylic acid (as in Capricin) is a fatty acid derived from coconuts and found in appreciable quantities in mother's milk. It can selectively inhibit the overgrowth of intestinal yeasts such as candida, yet does not adversely affect other 'friendly' microflora. Other benefits include a reduction in platelet stickiness, and a reduction in liver and plasma cholesterol content according to current data on Caprylic acid. Capricin also supplies highly available calcium and magnesium. It should be accompanied by acidophilus etc. supplementation in order to restore the balance in the intestinal flora. Research shows that a four-week course can often clear the intestines of candida, although a further course may be required prophylactically.

Hydrogen peroxide (H_2O_2) infusions or pills (said not to be so efficient) has been used to inactivate the fungal poisons in the blood and other poisons produced by viruses and bacteria, but there may be side effects from this treatment.

Garlic kills bacteria such as salmonella and *E. coli* and any fungal infection such as candida; should you object to garlic in food, take three capsules twice a day after meals, or use a liquid like Kyolic which is a very strong form of garlic concentrate. Allicin, the main anti-infective component of garlic, is now available in capsule form.

Poke root herb is said to be a specific.

Candida homoeopathic nosode 200 C can be taken once a week, or 30 C taken daily. (This is used routinely by homoeopaths.)

Iscador contains various regenerative muco-polypeptides. (It also contains the metal germanium, which has been found to help the subatomic particles in cells to 'spin' the correct way, whereas those in cancer cells spin the wrong way.) It is available in drops from Weleda, although it is normally given by injection, when it is considered to be more effective. It:

- Acts as an immune activator for cell wall repair.
- May have to be kept up for five years as a maintenance dose.
- Increases T lymphocytes.
- Helps breathing and haemoglobin count.
- Has a protective effect during chemotherapy or radiotherapy.

Avoid stress, which encourages stomach secretions which destroy the helpful bacteria.

Once candida levels have been reduced it is necessary to repair the damaged mucous membranes of the intestines through taking:

- Zinc.
- Vitamin B5 (calcium pantothenate).
- Vitamin E.

To help the immune system recover from the deleterious effects of PCC there are other measures that can be taken which may possibly require a change in lifestyle:

- Ensure that your house is not damp and producing mould; check particularly when symptoms are worse in damp muggy weather.
- Get out into natural light as much as possible.
- Exercise to stimulate circulation and respiration.
- Avoid stress; relax and meditate.
- Have no antibiotics, steroids or contraceptive pill for an extended period.

The object of preventative action is to influence the environment round the cells so that their walls are repaired. Swift detoxification is therefore required. The long-term objective is to try and stimulate the immune system.

ANTI-CANDIDA DIET

To begin with, eliminate:

- Food containing or derived from yeasts or fungi or gluten.
- Mushrooms.
- Yeast-containing foods such as Marmite, most stock cubes, beef extracts.
- Bread, breadcrumbs, cakes, biscuits, pasta. Note that gluten is in wheat, rye, oats (but oatbran is all right) and barley, but is not in rice, millet, corn (maize) or buckwheat.
- All vinegars, including apple cider vinegar.
- All fermented drinks, beers, spirits, wine, cider, etc.
- All malted products.
- Monosodium glutamate, found in many processed foods.
- All cheeses, particularly blue cheeses like Danish blue and gorgonzola.
- Dried fruits; stale nuts.
- Any pills which are yeast based, e.g. brewers yeast tablets.
- Any food containing sugar in any form, including honey, sweets, chocolate, soft drinks, etc., for at least three months (saccharine is permissible).

If possible, avoid the following:

- Foods with colourings, preservatives or additives.
- The whites of eggs which often have a lot of mould toxins.
- Pasteurised milk and beef because cattle are often fed on mouldy hay or grain. Lamb or wildfowl would be better.
- Mucus-forming foods, e.g. mueslis which have a large amount of yeasts which form extra mucus, dairy products.
- Gluten in wheat, rye, oats and barley, all of which form excessive mucus. Gluten behaves in the body very much like human protein but it has heavier and denser molecular characteristics. It is often found as a thickening agent of the walls of veins and arteries.

Instead you should eat the following:

- High-fibre diet. Take extra fibre (oatbran and oatgerm or psyllium husks, which are a source of non-allergenic fibre) to help accelerate elimination from bowels, 1–3 tsps in 8 oz water, increasing over 3–4 weeks to provide the extra fibre required.
- Protein such as fish (not smoked, and preferably deepwater fish), meat (not cured or salted, and preferably non-steroid fed).

- Mainly tropical fruits, not easily contaminated, such as kiwi, grapefruit, papaya.
- Millet, rice, maize, oatbran, pea flour, banana flour, buckwheat, but not soya. Porridge produces too much mucus which an ill person cannot break down. Porridge made of millet and oatbran is quite acceptable.
- Brown rice, which is far better than white.
- Yolks of eggs (not raw).
- Nuts and seeds that have been soaked overnight; pulses; sprouted seeds (lentil sprouts are very good). Any pulses or beans should always be soaked until they just begin to sprout; never eat them just boiled, because then the enzymes within them are destroyed allowing toxic chemicals to become inorganic and to generate harmful free radicals. One suggestion is to mash them and add them at the very last moment to a casserole, otherwise they become fairly indigestible. Once protein has been denatured it is not digested well; any beans that do not sprout are very indigestible.
- Vegetables of the brassica family, e.g. cabbages, kale, turnips, broccoli, cauliflower, brussel sprouts, radishes, mustard. Eat them raw or steamed.
- Lapacho (or taheebo) tea (Argentinian only recommended) which contains lapachel, a quinone, which is also very effective against cancers (especially leukaemia). There are a number of herbal compounds which are very potent as cleansers and detoxifiers.
- It is useful to liquidise seeds and nuts, which give very good highly digestible proteins, particularly linseed, sunflower and pumpkin seeds.
- Coffee will exacerbate stress on the emotional, physical and mental planes. Coffee is meant to be a diuretic, but if you burn it and store it in a jar, then it helps retain fluids and has no diuretic effect. If you have black coffee it stimulates the nerve endings; it also can help digestion, if taken without milk or sugar.
- A good quality wine, not fermented with added yeast and sugar, contains a high level of digestive enzymes. Organic wines are generally acceptable as they are cooled and not heat-treated (most wines are normally heat-treated). QMP on German wines means there is no added sugar. A little wine is all right as a treat, but arthritics should abstain.

It is important to try and help the immune system as much as possible with:

- An increase of oxygen supplies to cells (despite the fact that candida is an aerobic organism and requires oxygen to exist) with foods like garlic (whole or in pill form), onions, and metals such as germanium (found in garlic and *Aloe vera* particularly, and also in Iscador.

- Vitamin C in large quantities to counter the effect of chemical toxins (acetaldehyde particularly) produced by candida.
- Vitamins A (as beta-carotene), F (evening primrose oil), E and B5, especially if there are any allergies.
- Selenium.
- Zinc.
- Magnesium orotate.
- Biotin and/or oleic acid as in olive oil to stop the candida yeast changing into its more dangerous fungal form.
- L-arginine, an amino acid, at the start of any anti-candida campaign.
- Linseed oil for its linolenic acid which helps clear the intestines of fat and cholesterol and allows nutrients to be absorbed properly.
- Enzymes such as CoQ10 and pancreatic enzymes.
- Homoeopathic *Viscum album* is said to stimulate the thymus gland and restore normal enzyme and hormone metabolism.

Avoid stress as much as possible as it encourages stomach secretions which will destroy the 'helpful' bacteria in the gut. And exercise as much as possible (except patients with ME) and get out into the fresh air.

Finally, some general points relating to an anti-candida diet:

- Marinate foods with anti-fungal elements, e.g. lemon, garlic, onions, cinnamon, cloves, ginger, yoghourt.
- Chew all food well to allow enzymes in the saliva to break it down.
- Heavily roasted foods are bad; lightly grilled or roasted foods are very much better.
- Sprinkle a little cold-pressed oil mixed with water in a pan, then toss vegetables and bring up the heat. This will result in less oxidation of the food.
- There must be a complete breakdown of components of food, therefore only eat things which are easily broken down in the digestive process.
- Apples, pears, oranges and grapes all have yeast mould toxins, therefore eat mainly tropical fruits; for instance you can liquidise avocados, kiwifruit, pineapples, and then add acidophilus or yoghourt.
- Drink a little at a time, but often.

- Deepwater fish are safe to eat, but resist the temptation to eat fresh-water fish, which are often contaminated with bacteria and yeast compounds.
- Note that indoor commercially produced, and particularly prepacked, lettuces contain a high level of nitrates and are therefore a possible source of contamination.

15
MUCUS

Every time one takes mucus-forming foods, such as dairy products, more and more mucus is formed and deposited on the walls of the digestive organs, causing thick decaying matter to interfere with the metabolic function. The villi which transfer the nutrients from the gut into the bloodstream get flattened with this mucus debris and are therefore unable to accomplish their task – it is always an indication that excessive mucus is being produced whenever we cannot assimilate food properly. This becomes obvious when a person loses weight, despite having a healthy appetite and diet. This mucus build-up encourages colonisation and invasion of pathogenic bacteria, fungi and viruses into the digestive tract.

Many people have a continuous production of surplus mucus; when they get up in the morning they have a build-up of catarrh and phlegm in the back of their throat and nose for the first half hour in the morning. Many have post-nasal drip and congestion. Over-production of leucocytes is the initiator of this build-up of catarrh. The problem is that mucus is a medium ready to be colonised; it can be inoculated by any microorganisms such as staphylococci, candida species, *E. coli*, Tubercular bacilli and pneumococci. When there are any airborne microbes, such as in transmittable diseases, they too begin to infiltrate the mucus material.

However, yeast colonisation is the primary factor in any infections of mucus, other infections developing in the mucus which the yeast organisms have penetrated.

FORMATION OF MUCUS

It is important to know how mucus is formed, apart from milk and other dairy products. Concentrated proteins like meat, cheese or eggs are very dense and encourage mucus formation. These foods have been staple foods for many years and people cannot imagine that there might be something wrong with them. But denatured (cooked) dense proteins are not easily digestible. They are only all right if they carry some living enzymes which help with their digestion once they enter the body.

Generally modern foods have already been cooked or heat-treated, sterilised, prepared, frozen, reheated, etc., and have had all the enzymes in them destroyed. The protein chains and fatty acids are therefore tightly packed and carry no self-digesting enzymes. We ingest the proteins and fats and try to degrade them in our stomach, but without the enzymes and other factors which are essential to help in the breakdown of those proteins and fats. These denatured food particles, instead of being digested in the stomach properly, then carry on into the small intestine undegraded (undigested), and from there they get into the bloodstream through the action of microorganisms such as candida, *E. coli*, etc., which allow undigested proteins to filter through into the blood. The gut-blood barrier of filters and immunosurveillance activity thus collapses.

It is this mechanism which we have to overcome when ill. In particular such ailments as colitis, irritable bowel syndrome, enterocolitis, and coeliac conditions are an indication that there is a great amount of inflammation in the gut, particularly in the small intestines, as well as large amounts of mucus deposits infected by pathogens and other toxins.

A pseudo-intestinal wall, which is really a thick coating of mucus and fibrous material, made up of live and dead bacteria, fungus and enteroviruses, is built up. Once they have died back they do not always disappear but stay as dead matter, then calcify and harden, building up a lining of pseudo-tissue plastered against the true intestinal wall. Here there will thrive a high number of unpleasant organisms. The phenomenon of unwanted proliferation of foreign matter in the blood shows as fibrositis in cystic fibrosis or fibrosis in fibroids. Arteriosclerosis, multiple sclerosis, mucopolysaccharide disease, etc., are differing stages of the same process of gathering of mucus and toxins in different organs and systems.

Fungus is made up primarily of protein, hormones, calcium and sugar and becomes fibrous very quickly. The life cycle of fungi is very short. They come into being quickly, take over the tissues, colonise, excrete like all living organisms, producing byproducts called mycotoxins. High temperatures, such as those reached during the baking of bread, will not affect these mycotoxins, which can still retain their toxic characteristics above 400°F. These mycotoxins can insiduously break down the immune system, because they are very similar in structure chemically and biochemically to our own mucoproteins and hormones. The body does not therefore see them as strangers or invaders; they are allowed to get through, bypass the surveillance system of the body, and become part of the bonding structure of our own proteins, even getting right into the cell nuclei and causing disturbances in the genetic material, whose species' identity is then lost.

Mycotoxins are not only contaminants that cause tissue damage but are teratogenic (i.e. affect all creatures and all species and are therefore non-species-related). They are also genetic mutants, disturbing genetic pools and causing severe genetic mutations. Many disease processes such as bacterial, fungal and viral infections may evolve into more complex life-forms – especially that of the mycotic biological chemical entities, which are among the most aggressive cancer-inducing substances known to man. Under certain circumstances, where there are toxic substances like radium and some heavy metals, instead of dying back, they further decompose into highly toxic compounds. Heavy metals can also encourage the mutation of organisms because they alter their metabolic electrolytic properties, and can, for example, encourage a microorganism which is normally an airborne entity, to become a macroorganism which can grow limbs or root systems, adapting to the conditions in the growing medium, thus becoming a mycellium.

However, not all yeasts become mycellia, and not all yeasts become bacteria; they are only able to do so when the right materials allow for their free radical colonisation. Elements such as sulphur, aluminium, caesium, strontium, lead, or mercury, by generating faulty combustion of biochemical and chemical compounds, encourage the evolution of pathogenic organisms.

Mucus is thus made up of undigested proteins, fats and muco-secretions from metabolic waste. Good bacteria break down mucoproteins into components for blood and tissue regeneration. When cooking eggs, for example, their substance becomes denatured before it enters the body and it will then be pounced on by the 'bad' bacteria (pathogens) which digest denatured food; they go for the already-decomposing material, such as protein that has been heat-treated or cooked, which has no enzyme life. Where minerals have been separated, vitamins have been broken down, protein has been destroyed, fats have been oxidised, the food is already decomposed, chemically speaking, as all its components have been separated beforehand. When someone eats eggs, for instance, and does produce mucus it means the undegraded mucoprotein is passing on to other areas of the body.

When there is mucus over-production it is a sign that the body is trying to throw off toxins. It is the protective mechanism which is making our mucous membranes oversecrete mucus. Until there is a cleansing of the gastrointestinal system and regeneration of tissue in the alimentary canal we are going to be shifting mucus around, not for months, but years. Up to a third of body weight of a sick person may be foreign mucoproteins lodged in different parts of the body, which have to be expelled somehow in order to regain health.

If the food we eat also contains a high level of mucus-forming substances, there will be many foreign mucoproteins in the foodball, so the body has a problem recognising and identifying what is human, plant, animal or microbial protein. However, if one eats in such a manner that the body does not generate mucus-forming responses, e.g. by starting a meal with something raw, then the body will produce the necessary digestive enzymes and acids to digest completely any food taken in and convert it into easily assimilable healthy nutrients.

Any food that has been denatured, e.g. pasteurised, cooked or baked, makes the body produce white cells (leucocytes) very rapidly. Mucus-producing hot food, especially denatured proteins, immediately accelerates the production of leucocytes. Mucus is formed straight away in the throat, trachea and oesophagus. By the time the foodball gets to the stomach it is totally surrounded by and embedded in mucus, which becomes a barrier of elastic and sticky matter, not easily degradable when infiltrated by foreign proteins. In the stomach we do not have the necessary juices to break down this highly complex range of mucroproteins, so they stay there longer than they should. The food is then food for the fungi and bacteria and not for the host; there will be no absorption of properly broken down components of any real nutritive value which could provide the building blocks for healthy blood and tissue.

LEUCOCYTOSIS

If there is a lot of catarrh, then the body is overproducing white cells (leucocytosis); streaming catarrh is an indication that the body is producing a high level of leucocytes, the basis of mucus formation. This has the effect of slowing down lymph material, leading to a thick mucus formation. The ensuing catarrh of the chest will inhibit the functioning of the thymus gland.

Catarrh is a fibrous material and chronic catarrh results in the glands becoming embedded in dry mucus which forms a kind of fibrous chain which at times becomes stone hard, e.g. stones in the bladder, kidney or gallbladder, where the mucus is dried up and impacted. It may take years for the mucus inside our bodies to solidify, and it will therefore take months to shift it.

Even yoghourt – being milk – will bring on mucus production, but it may be preferable to carry on with yoghourt so that one knows that beneficial bacteria are colonising the gut, as opposed to mucus-forming pathogens. Furthermore, too many leucocytes are produced in response to any heated or degraded food. For example, in the early morning mucous membranes have microorganism residues, and if you take a cup of tea hot then immediately your membranes will produce a lot more lymphocytes, which will form a high level of mucus secretions that wraps up the microorganisms that are cultured on the mucous membranes; the result is that you have catarrh, with much more mucus on the whole of the trachea and oesophagus.

Leucocytosis is one precursor to all degenerative diseases involving the metabolism of proteins, because it puts the body into a phase of over-production of mucus which then feeds microorganisms. It also slows down the whole digestive process and retards the production of digestive enzymes which should be generated when we eat or drink anything raw or live. This is avoidable by taking, say, a glass of mineral water, with lemon or vitamin C, a glass of vegetable juice, *crudités* or salad before meals; in this way you reduce the production of a high level of leucocytes. Have a cold juice start to a breakfast and then have a cup of tea; the membranes will then be acclimatised to the nature of the food coming in. When we start with something hot then the production of mucus is much higher, thus slowing down digestion. Even if one has porridge it is possible to have a glass of mineral water or vegetable juice first. Therefore start all meals, always, with something raw to prepare the membranes for the subsequent breakdown of the more indigestible materials. This will generate the production of the HCL and digestive enzymes needed for the digestion of more coarse and complex food. A sample meal could be avocado salad, with watercress, then fish with steamed vegetables, ending up with cheese and celery, or avocado and prawns to begin with, then a hot dish, ending up with yoghourt, avocado and kiwi fruit mousse – no need for any other sweetening. All the components will be digested much more easily than if you start with hot soup, another hot dish and end up with fruit or apple pie and cream. The former gives at least two hours' advantage in the digestion processes needed to break down proteins and fats.

If the gut is entirely contaminated with candida species or other microorganisms, then we are not capable of absorbing nutrients. The first measure therefore is to modify the flora of the gut. Every time we take in sugars (even minor amounts, such as a piece of chocolate or a sweet drink) we colonise large numbers of the wrong sorts of microorganisms, and every time this happens a lot of mucus is formed, with the result that the transportation of nutrients will take place in a faulty manner.

Children today often have the illnesses of old age because their tissues are laced with undigested toxic metabolic waste. Their damaged gut cannot transport the appropriate nutrients into the bloodstream, to ensure there is healthy growth.

To understand the concept that the small intestine is either the factory of death or the factory of life is quite alien to us. However we either cause our own demise through faulty eating and living or we can cleanse the pipelines and then get the villi and gut wall to work again so that we can absorb the nutrients required for health, in which case of course, we would not require any extra vitamins, minerals, tonics or other food supplements to be healthy; pills of nutrients can never replace the wonderful nutrients in real food.

16
GLUTEN

It is useful to examine the properties of some common foods so that people with a degenerative disease will know what to avoid, what can be eaten regularly and what can be eaten as a treat sometimes. Any flatulence and dyspepsia means that the food eaten is not being rightly assimilated. The wrong food will feed and therefore help to colonise the wrong microorganisms in the digestive organs. In considering an eating plan for cancer sufferers, one major change to normal eating habits is to cut down on any products that have gluten in them.

Gluten is a very tough, very sticky, transparent, viscous substance when transported by and assimilated into the blood and the lymph, making them thick and morbid. Gluten, affecting the nature of our body fluids and mucoproteins, has a structure alien to the body metabolism; it sticks to anything and encapsulates smaller molecules such as sugar, cholesterol, fats, or salts, which are then transported into the blood as such, inefficiently digested. Byproducts of gluten get into the blood very quickly, especially through a damaged gut, even within an hour. A healthy person has a strong lining to the gut and a healthy bacterial flora within it, so many of the gluten particles will be eliminated through the faeces. But when a person is sick and the gut is very porous, gluten's main means of transportation is through the small intestine; from there it goes to other organs such as the liver, spleen, pancreas or gallbladder, causing disturbances in the functions of those organs, and it becomes embedded in the tissues throughout the organism. Gluten in modern grain strains is the major interfering factor in all the digestive processes, more so than many other substances especially in the early period of life – babyhood, childhood and adolescence.

Gluten enters the blood as if it were a true protein, but it is an invasive foreign one. Our body of course needs protein, as found in all grains, but the modern glutenous compounds are deleterious because they are not easily degradable, their molecular weight and density is so high that they succeed in imitating human protein chains, but they are totally different in molecular performance.

In response to a severe allergen, as gluten is, the body produces very high numbers of white blood cells (leucocytes) as a protective allergic response. Leucocytes are whitish, elastic and very similar in structure to gluten, and between the two they produce a thick mucus-like substance which envelopes the foodball, resulting in practically undigestible protein bonds. Where there are fungal, bacterial, or viral organisms growing in the gut, the first thing they will digest will be the mucoproteins surrounding the foodball, causing excretions of metabolic waste.

When the small intestine is full of this sticky gungey mucus, the 'good' bacteria are not going to survive in such an alkaline environment and the whole of the small intestine gets colonised with *Candida albicans* and other pathogens. This common yeast/mould then grows and overwhelms remaining useful bacteria. What then happens is poor digestion of foods, with the result that the host is not getting properly nourished.

Gluten is present in the bodies of modern people to such a high degree that, in some instances, it makes up about one-fifth of the total body weight. It is present in the joints, over nerve tissues in the form of fibroids, etc., and a lot of gluten will have been dispersed through the blood to many tissues of the body. Westerners especially are so used to living on bread, biscuits, pasta, muesli, etc., that glutenous grain make for the bulk of their food intake.

There may be, for instance, a joint problem, for example arthrosis. If we have an infiltration of microorganisms via the blood or lymph, and the sedimentation rate is high in the interstitial fluid in the joints, possibly as a result of being invaded by glutenous and other residual compounds, free radical damage will occur, then necrosis in the bone as well as in the cartilage will ensue. Yet, for this arthrosis to evolve, first of all we must have degeneration of the small intestine, i.e. the gateway to the bloodstream must be open. The first line of defence therefore is to consider what is reaching the target organs or systems via this route. The primary action to take is to cleanse the small intestine first, together with the colon, otherwise the blood will be carrying byproducts, allergens, gluten, etc., to already weakened tissues, wherever the weakness may be.

Gluten nowadays is not the same as it was prior to about 1900 because it was then that hybridisation of cereals started. Prior to that time, gluten protein in wheat had totally different characteristics and living systems had developed the processes needed to modify and break down that form of protein completely. Since the war the big millers and producers have produced specific strains of wheat designed for better grading and baking qualities yet possessing altered genetic and biological characteristics.

GLUTEN AND DISEASE

It is necessary to recognise gluten for what it is. It is not necessarily a threat. It will not be life threatening as long as we are capable of taking measures that are truly corrective. We can excise a tumour, but part of the process must be for the individual to undergo a period of detoxification and real change in their lives so that corrective measures can be taken to inhibit further developments of this kind. Treatment may be by chemotherapy, which poisons the tumour cells but may spread toxic material into other parts of the body; when a culturing medium exists elsewhere in the body the process is bound to start again. A recent study of over 700 elderly people found they had had many tumours (up to 20 metastases) of which they were unaware, but they lived a normal life, probably through having a strong immune system right up until death. Furthermore, in a study of American soldiers who had died:

- During the First World War, only 5 per cent aged between 22 and 30 had degeneration of the arteries (arteriosclerosis).
- At the end of the Second World War this had risen to 52 per cent.
- By the time of the Vietnam war it had risen further to 95 per cent!

This is therefore a very new phenomenon in the history of mankind, brought about by changes in agriculture, the hybridisation and genetic engineering of plants and animals, and the genetic manipulation of human material by the use of contraceptives and hormone therapy which often conflicts with systemic function. Gluten plus fungi, and pathogenic secretions, are the main stressors of tissues.

Cancers in the maize-eating populations are very low (only where hygiene is poor are there some cancers of the gullet), especially where grain management is still correct, with good storage, no hybridisation and proper growing and ripening. In a recent study in Canada and the United States on 236 stillborn babies with no actual visible cause of death, it was found that up to one-third of their body weight contained toxic metabolites, of which:

- Gluten was 53 per cent.
- Cow's milk byproducts, transferred through the placenta, were 27 per cent.
- Mould, bacterial and viral residues were 20 per cent.

Of these babies, 171 had so much lingering sticky glutenous material that their organs could not function. Functional seizures are very common in infants (e.g. cot deaths). They had constantly been receiving toxic residues in the womb which they just could not cope with or process adequately. These toxins were foreign mucoproteins, pesticides and pollutants, which had congealed in their bodies and had interpenetrated all their organs, even though outwardly they were perfectly normal. Every system in the body had antigenically foreign mucus material in it; every organ had been invaded by mucoproteins foreign to the baby, mucoprotein which was not true to the mother's protein but consisted of animal, plant, fungal and bacterial protein – not human protein at all. Many of them had tumours or cysts. The mixture of animal and plant proteins, fats, sugars and chelated toxins make up multiple molecules; they in turn make clusters, and the lymph glands cannot drain off this solidified or emulsified alien cellular matter.

Gluten sensitivity or gluten intolerance shows up as dyspepsia, a lot of abdominal rumblings, the digestion not really working well, oedema, a feeling of being tired all the time, gritty eyes. Many coeliacs (who must never eat food with gluten in it) are also intolerant of milk, and there would appear to be a relationship between milk and gluten intolerances, especially when the animals are fed with grains. Gluten intolerance may, in fact, by a sequel to milk intolerance in childhood.

Degenerative diseases appear when gluten is not being broken down properly. A number of research units worldwide have shown clearly that when material is tagged with radioisotopes, particles of gluten can be seen in the bloodstream less than two hours after ingestion. It is therefore a very fast process, which occurs only after the gut lining has become diseased.

- Multiple sclerosis – there appears to be a reasonably strong correlation between the incidence of multiple sclerosis and the consumption of glutenous grains and denatured proteins and fats.
- Rheumatoid arthritis – similarly, a person may be more likely to contract rheumatoid arthritis where he is suffering from malabsorption of nutrients due to the action of gluten and toxic remnants of metabolic waste.
- Schizophrenia – it has been shown that byproducts of gluten and other toxins may enter the brain tissue and disturb it, as can be surmised from the fact that coeliacs often become schizophrenic, their mental disturbances disappearing after they are put on a gluten-free low toxic load diet. Gluten has been found to have crossed the blood-brain barrier in schizophrenic patients, thus interfering with neurological command messages, with hormonal metabolism and with nutrient assimilation.

Anywhere where there is tissue damage there is an indication of poor combustion of toxic waste. Gluten makes it worse; it is not itself a carcinogen, but it makes a kind of film over the tissue and therefore inhibits the pick-up mechanism of oxygen as well as the modification and repair which should take place by the natural movement of the principal repair agents; if they cannot get to the trouble spot, because of the wrong mucoproteins which have coated the tissue, it is much more difficult to get the repair job done. For example, with MS, people who are on a gluten-free, fat-free, toxins-reduced diet plus supplements make reasonable progress, as it is believed that gluten interrupts the flow of messages through the nerves due to its glue-like characteristics. In lymphoedema a gluten-free diet will significantly increase the flow of lymph fluids, and patients quickly show an improvement in lymph drainage. A change in diet, coupled with other therapies such as physiotherapy, can therefore help enormously.

GLUTEN AND DIET

It is the current thinking that people should eat more fibre, but in wheat fibre there are particles of bran in which there are gluten and fungal proteins and very high levels of environmental toxins like heavy metals and even radioactive compounds. So, although the wheat fibre is important, it is undesirable in other ways, and it is suitable only as an occasional treat.

In British or Canadian wheats there is now between 12–15 per cent gluten, which has a much higher molecular weight and density than a human protein. Gluten has the ability to wrap itself round other molecules, and is almost an 'imposter', imitating the human or animal proteins and competing with them in the synthesis of different elements of tissue requirements.

Any microorganisms in the gut should be participating in the process of digestion, alongside the acids and enzymes. When the microorganisms glut on the surface gluten material, or on leucocytes, they thrive in the wrong areas (trachea, oesophagus) and do not allow digestion to take place properly. Food therefore goes undigested (e.g. corn on the cob, seeds, grains, vegetables can often be seen in the faeces having passed through undigested), as a result of the mucoproteins adhering to and coating the walls of the stomach and the foodball. The food will then be feeding the bacterial or fungal cultures and the nutrients will not be going into the bloodstream to enable the building up of healthy tissues and organs.

What will eventually get into the bloodstream will be partly undigested proteins, sugars and toxic waste. These toxins have to be disposed of; failing that, they are deposited in the weakest spots – where there are probably already microorganisms ready and waiting for food. Toxic waste then helps these microorganisms to grow and proliferate in a given area. Gradually they will make inroads in any area where there is undigested food still not completely broken down into the building blocks – the amino acids, sugars fats, vitamins, minerals and metals – required by the body to sustain a healthy life.

For example, fats will stick and oxidise inside veins, heart and arteries, etc.; gluten sticks to cholesterol, which is fixed by the gluten molecule to the tissue. There is no danger from cholesterol if there is no gluten available to fix it. Peroxidated fat molecules are attached and engulfed by the very large gluten molecules, which also wrap themselves round many other smaller molecules.

New scientific findings suggest that no foods containing gluten should be given to babies in the first year of life, to protect the lining of the gut. After that they can cope better with denatured foods; otherwise they absorb mucoproteins not of human origin into their blood, right from the start.

Anyone with a degenerative disease or a disabling all-pervading chronic illness will have a damaged gut that enables the transportation of material, which may be toxic, from the gut into the blood. This transportation mechanism we cannot stop unless we stop ingesting the material that is likely to generate toxic waste, i.e. we cannot stop the allergic process unless we stop ingesting the offending materials. There are plenty of other foods to have, which mean we do not need to go on a very restrictive diet.

Gluten is in wheat, rye, oats and barley, but not in millet, rice or most types of corn, although even some rice and maize, through hybridisation, have now been made glutenous. Oatbran and oatgerm, on the other hand, are almost free of gluten as the gluten is in the centre of the oats. One should not eat wheat, rye, oats or barley unless as sprouted grains, particularly as there is the double danger of gluten, fungus and pollutant residues which greatly increase the contamination with foreign proteins and hormones. In sprouting seeds the gluten protein is reprocessed in the sprouting process. It is really within our control whether or not we eat foods containing gluten, and it should be appreciated that if there is an active malignancy, wheat and glutenous grains should only be eaten as an occasional treat. It will always be safest to choose foods that are not contaminated by fungi and/or gluten to reduce the toxic load. (Note that monosodium glutamate [MSG, E 621] is derived from gluten; if eating out you should ask for food that has no MSG, even at Chinese restaurants.)

When eating any form of wheat flour one is taking in about 15 per cent gluten protein and plant hormones which are not easily degradable. Some will be expelled as mucus, some via the bowels or through the skin (acne, eczema, boils, etc.), but there is still very much left behind as hardening, sclerotic material. Wheat is the most toxic glutenous grain, and many modern hybrid grains are particularly glutenous.

Grains are a marvellous food and once used to provide the main building blocks in nutrients for the body. But now it is different. Healthy people can take some wheat, their immune responses and healthy flora in the gut keeping fungi and gluten in check. But when the body is storing a lot of protein compounds, especially gluten, the results are the modern epidemics of herpes, candida, thrush and other more serious degenerative diseases. People born at the turn of the century had their bodies formed by food in its original natural form, but since the advent of hybridisation and pasteurisation things have changed. Of course a small amount of bread will not hurt anyone, but it is the constant taking in of glutenous substances that does cause long-term damage problems.

PRACTICAL MEASURES FOR GLUTEN-FREE FOOD

It should be emphasised that where a person is demonstrably gluten-intolerant it is important to adhere to a gluten-free diet for life. Having said that, it is appreciated that it is almost impossible to avoid all gluten as it is so often hidden in manufactured products or is taken indirectly through eating meat or fish from animals that have been fed on grains.

In a Good Health Guide, *Gluten Intolerance* (issued by Keats Publishing), there is a recipe for home-made baking powder that can be made from gluten-free grains. Blend together 3 ounces of a tolerated flour with 2 ounces of cream of tartar, 2 ounces of tartaric acid and 2½ ounces of bicarbonate of soda. Sift all the ingredients twice through a flour sieve. Store the blend in a tightly closed airtight container.

Millet gluten-free bread is worth trying. Here is a recipe:

250 g of millet flour
290 ml (just under half a pint) of water
2 tbsp of ground almonds
½ tsp salt
2 tsp of gluten-free baking powder
2 tbsp of sesame oil

First make a starchy paste. Add 30 g (about 2 level tbsp) of the flour to 250 ml (9 fl oz) of the water in a non-stick pan, stir vigorously and heat gently. The paste will gradually thicken. Keep stirring and don't let it burn. When it is smooth and fairly thick it will take on a translucent look. Take off the heat and let it cool, giving it an occasional stir.

While it cools, add the baking powder to another 40 ml (just under 2 fl oz) of water at bloodheat, plus 2 tbsp ground almonds. Stir and leave in a warm place until a nice creamy head has risen on it – about 15–30 minutes. By this time your starch paste should be cool.

Add the rest of the flour and the salt to the starch paste, and stir in well. Then add the baking powder and the oil, stir for five minutes (the equivalent to kneading). Don't expect an elastic dough; what you should have is a very thick, heavy batter, too thick to pour. If it's too dense, add a little more lukewarm water or goat's milk.

Grease a small bread tin – ideally the batter should half fill it – with vegetable oil, scrape in the batter with a spatula, smooth over the top, cover with a clean damp tea towel and leave to rise in a warm place until the batter has doubled in bulk – about 3–4 hours. Then bake in an oven pre-heated to 400°F/210°C/gas mark 6 for 40–45 minutes, until brown and hollow-sounding on top. Turn out on to a wire rack and leave to cool for at least eight hours.

Note: the amount of water will vary according to the grain used. Study the batter each time you bake a loaf to see which degree of thickness gave the best results. And if the loaf tends to be a little soft and moist on the bottom, just upend it and pop it back into the still-hot oven for five minutes.

In the fibre of many wheats there are often present fungal protein and hormones, as well as gluten, so wholemeal bread has almost double the amount of toxins compared with white bread. Although wholemeal has the most nutrient value, it has the most permeable and the most contaminated bran. So, to minimise the amount of trigger factors in any condition where degenerative changes are taking place in the body, it is better to go for a white flour product than a wholemeal product once in a while. Instead use oatbran and germ, psyllium husks and linseed (Linusit) for your dietary fibre unless you can find producers who can ensure a supply of safe grains.

Ryvita has far less gluten than wheat, but it still has some, so have it only as a treat, in rotation with corn and rice perhaps. Use corn flour as a substitute for wheat flour as often as possible. There may be a small amount of fungal toxins in corn when milled, but it is only in the 'heart' of the corn, whereas in wheat the fungal toxins will be found all round the seed, and on the surface area of the outside of the wheat which is contaminated by pollutants and air-borne organisms.

17
FREE RADICALS

A cell can be visualised as a poached egg shape with the nucleus (the yolk) full of chromosomes (the genetic material). All the time there are toxins invasively attacking the cell wall. Carcinogens are those toxins that manage to pierce the cell wall, attack the nucleus and split its chromosomes giving birth to oncogenes. This destruction of the cells results in the formation of rogue molecules called free radicals, which are released, and also in the advent of gene material which then attempts to form cells, although in this case the cells are not normal and do not obey the normal cycles of cell reproduction.

WHAT ARE FREE RADICALS?

- They are molecules which are out of balance. Each molecule in the body has a cloud of electrons spinning round it. A free radical is a molecule which has gained, or lost, an electron and is therefore unbalanced and unstable, with an impaired electron in its outer orbit.
- They are cell-damaging toxins; by stealing electrons from balanced molecules in the cell in order to bring themselves into balance, they weaken the cell considerably, which then dies. This process weakens tissues, then organs, then the body itself. In the process they create new free radicals, thus initiating a chain reaction of increasing numbers of free radicals, with a resultant increase in cell damage.
- Free radicals are the result of oxidation reactions such as the reaction of oxygen with some metals or polyunsaturated fatty acids (PUFAs), helped by radiations and/or ultraviolet light.
- They behave literally as spears, repeatedly piercing, puncturing and often severing complete portions of cells and cell walls; they can even destroy collagen fibres.
- They can result from eating certain foods and being exposed to certain chemicals which help in the formation of the free radical molecules which cause serious damage to cells, enzymes and genetic material such as DNA and RNA molecules, the very basis of life.

- Free radical molecules sometimes get so numerous that they overwhelm the body's ability to overcome them and the system breaks down at its weakest point.
- The damage may manifest itself as an inflamed joint, an infection, or a tumour. Inflammation is a result of free radical activity, e.g. arthritis or gout, when the synovial fluid in the joints lose their lubricating ability. Normally this 'joint oil' is kept healthy through the work of the catalase enzyme complex and SOD (superoxide dismutase).

The knowledge of the damage done by free radicals has only really been recognised in the last few years. It is now believed that this kind of process, by which free radicals split the atoms of oxygen, hydrogen or nitrogen, taking just one single atomic charge means that free radicals are the essential promoters of both cancer and all degenerative processes. This is further exacerbated by any form of stress.

If, on top of that, one has microorganisms multiplying in the presence of high levels of toxic residues, then one does not stand a chance – the more microorganisms multiply, the more toxic wastes they produce. It is a vicious circle. In cases of shock or prolonged stress, excessive adrenaline may be produced to counter the stress, but byproducts of this adrenaline also act as 'arrows' to split the oxygen atoms. Excessive adrenaline is thus a major toxic culprit in all degenerative diseases. Normally adrenaline is balanced with stamina and is a necessary hormone for flight or fight. However if one has too much of it in response to non-aggressive situations or emergencies, a lot is secreted, cannot perhaps be used and then has to be stored in the body. And it is the stored byproduct of glandular metabolism that becomes highly toxic when the free radical 'singlets' are produced.

HOW ARE FREE RADICALS FORMED?

A normal molecule is made up of atoms bonded together by pairs of electron 'bridges'. Sometimes (due to toxin attacks or carcinogens) the bonding breaks and a molecule with a single electron gets detached. This is a free radical. Each molecule in the body has pairs of electrons spinning round it. A free radical is a molecule which has gained, or lost, an electron and is therefore unbalanced and unstable. They are called 'free' because, having only one electron, this molecule cannot attach itself to other normal molecules which have two electrons. These free radicals thus become highly active and unstable and may then:

- 'Steal' a second electron from another normal molecule, making that molecule a free radical in its turn, as it only has one electron left. They are thus highly reactive chemical agents and can combine with anything that lingers around such as the toxic molecules of decaying mucoproteins and plant and animal proteins in the gut that have not been completely digested.
- 'Bump' into another free radical and join up to make a rogue molecule which can be an initiator of a disease process.
- Be attracted to free radical scavengers (such as vitamins A, E, C, beta-carotene, CoQ10, silymarin and SOD) which have extra spare electrons which they can give up without damage to themselves.

X-ray treatment or diagnosis can be very damaging as it produces large numbers of free radicals; despite large sums having been spent on the research for better diagnostic machines, the latest generation of X-ray diagnostic tool – the computerised tomography or CAT scanner – produces as many free radicals as its less sophisticated predecessors. Ultrasound also splits oxygen molecules, with the same result – the production of free radicals. Whenever possible you should therefore ask for diagnosis by nuclear magnetic resonance (NMR) imaging.

SUPEROXIDES

Oxygen is absolutely essential to all plants, animals and humans, as it reacts with so many different chemicals, e.g. combining haemoglobin in the red blood cells to produce oxyhaemoglobin; the bloodstream then carries the oxygen round the body, locked up in the red blood cells, delivering it to the cells and tissues where it fuels the various biochemical reactions.

Some free radicals are formed as normal byproducts of the metabolic use of oxygen and food nutrients to produce ATP (the basic energy storage molecule). These are oxygen molecules with unpaired electrons, and are called superoxides. The superoxides have an important role as they dissolve any invading foreign matter that the phagocytes or macrophages have absorbed. Provided there are sufficient naturally occurring antioxidant enzymes, such as catalase or superoxide dismutase (SOD), circulating in the body, then these superoxides are kept within control. (Note that these natural enzymes remove free radicals many times quicker than antioxidant nutrients (see below). Note also that when there is stress of any kind – chemical emotional, physical, infection – the production of superoxides is increased.)

Excess superoxides are extremely dangerous for normal cells, and it is thought that they are nearly always involved in the development of diseases; for example, proteins and nucleic acids (DNA and RNA, which carry the genetic blueprint which cells use to reproduce themselves) can be damaged, leading to the proliferation of abnormal cells, which can become cancers, or to an acceleration of the aging process.

Some superoxides are formed from a reaction with hydrogen and are called hydrogen peroxides. In turn, some free radicals, called hydroxyls, are formed from the reaction with a peroxide. (The only known enzyme that removes hydroxl radicals is methionine reductase, which is therefore essential where the hydroxyls have been formed by exposure to radiation.) The enzyme catalase helps the breakdown of hydrogen peroxide to water and free oxygen.

Some peroxides may also be created by the process of lipid peroxidation (fat oxidation) which is a contributory factor in the process of aging; they are peroxides (molecules with a harmful excess of oxygen) leading to oxygen toxicity which is responsible for injury to tissues in such ailments as arthritis, lupus, heart attacks, skin cancer, eczema, age spots, dermatitis, psoriasis, liver damage, as well as injury as a result of cancer chemotherapy drugs such as Adriamycin, which can itself lead to heart diseases. (Note that CoQ10 is said to reverse the toxic effects of Adriamycin and other anthracyclines rapidly.) It has also been found that the bioflavonoids of the *Gingko biloba* leaves scavenge hydroxyls and therefore prevent lipid peroxidation.

The maintenance of the correct balance of superoxides is a key to good health and longevity. Superoxide dismutase (SOD) is an enzyme that disperses superoxides. It is produced naturally in the body, but its production may tail off as one gets older, therefore allowing more superoxides to remain in the body. It has been conjectured that some people, possibly 5 per cent of the population, cannot secrete sufficient SOD naturally and they are therefore constitutionally more predisposed to developing cancer. Such people require antioxidants as prophylactics. SOD tends to get broken down in the digestive tract, but when it is liposomal-encapsulated (enteric coated) it is made available as an antioxidant.

The bloodstream carries nutrients round the body, and removes waste materials from the tissues and cells. This exchange of nutrients for waste products is carried out in the capillary vessels, a network of tiny blood vessels that permeates the whole body. An excess of superoxides will however impede the blood circulation and slow down the flow to the capillaries, possibly even coagulate the blood itself, and have a deleterious effect on organs and tissues – for example, the skin becomes less resilient and drier – all signs of aging. This constriction of the blood flow can lead to heart diseases or strokes, again more common in the aged.

WHAT DAMAGE CAN FREE RADICALS DO?

Free radicals are responsible for cell damage in every single degenerative disease. They have been found to be a factor aggravating diseases such as degenerative joint rheumatism, Crohn's disease, ulcerative colitis and multiple sclerosis. This is further exacerbated by any form of stress.

- They can damage the protective membranes of cells.
- They turn body lipids (fats) rancid, either hardening the cell membrane or puncturing it so that the cell collapses and the cell fluid drains out. This can be seen as a wrinkling of the skin.
- In joints the gritty toxins accumulate, causing friction, heat, swelling and eventual damage to the joint itself, as in arthritis, bursitis or gout.
- In the lymph fluid they lead to leukaemia.
- In the central nervous system they can lead to such diseases as motor neurone disease, myasthenia gravis, schizophrenia.
- They can get into the cells and damage their mitochondria (those parts of cells which provide the energy for cellular function).
- They can damage DNA and RNA in a cell's nucleus. As DNA is responsible for the exact reproduction of the cell, any damage to it will mean that abnormal cells will be formed and a chain reaction occurs, with more and more imperfect cells being produced, leading to disease and eventually death. These abnormal cells in turn trigger the immune system to attack such unnatural 'invaders', i.e. the body attacks itself (this is called an autoimmune disease).

It has been found that many people with cancer can live normally if they have a strong immune system. (In this regard the older generations are at an advantage, as newer generations are weaker due to things like anti-biotics directly administered on a wide scale or through the food chain.) Through a weakening of the immune system, and therefore an inability to eliminate superoxides, particularly in the elderly, there is an increased risk of their succumbing to ailments that they would normally be able to fight. By controlling free radicals we thus slow the ageing process. New cells are being created all the time, but after our 20s more cells die than are created, and the aging process begins. Many cells are killed, unnecessarily, by free radical damage, and this accelerates the aging process.

HOW DOES THE BODY COPE WITH FREE RADICALS?

Under normal conditions the body can cope with these free radicals, keeping them in check by a complex of natural antioxidant enzymes called SOD (superoxide dismutase), glutathione peroxidase, methionine reductase and catalase. But when we age, or when we do not receive adequate nutrition, this production of natural antioxidant enzymes decreases.

Furthermore, it must be pointed out that some free radicals are used by our white blood cells to destroy dangerous substances in a very selective and specific manner.

HOW CAN FREE RADICALS BE KEPT UNDER CONTROL OR ELIMINATED?

Principally by the use of antioxidants which are able to slow down, if not prevent, certain free radical-forming processes. Antioxidants are therefore also anti-cancer agents, because the chemical reactions that lead to the formation of dangerous free radicals (the causative factors in many cancers) need oxygen. Useful antioxidants are:

- Vitamin C is the most important antioxidant. It can prevent the transformation of nitrates into cancerous nitrosamines. It also helps against cancers caused by ultraviolet rays, and certain chemical pollutants such as benzopyrene. It can be given as an intravenous drip, plus micronutrients, or as a supplement. It is useful to spray any fruit or vegetables that have been cut or chopped with a solution of, say, 1 gram of vitamin C to half a pint of water.
- Vitamin A and beta-carotene (pro-vitamin A) inhibit cancers of the skin, provoked by ultraviolet rays such as acquired by too much sunbathing, as well as various gastrointestinal cancers. Up to 50,000 iu per day can be taken under supervision, but do not exceed this dose. Beta-carotene is a highly active free radical scavenger.
- Vitamin E (α tocopherol) reduces the production of free radicals from PUFAs and prevents formation of nitrosamines. Take up to a maximum of 800 iu per day, but start low at about 250 iu. Both vitamins A and E boost the body's synthesis of CoQ10, a powerful antioxidant itself.
- Enzymes such as SOD (which removes the most common free radical, i.e. superoxides) must be used together with catalase (which removes hydrogen peroxide from the tissues). SOD needs to be enteric coated to allow it to pass through the acidity of the stomach and be broken down in the alkaline medium of the small

intestine. To be most effective it needs to be part of an enzyme complex, with selenium, vitamins A, C and E, glutathione peroxidase and CoQ10, as well as catalase. Through its ability to maintain health and prevent aging, SOD can be used as a preventive medicine.

- Silymarin is prepared from the fruit of *Carduus marianus* (milk thistle) and has a specific action on the liver.
- Amino acids such as cysteine, methionine and glutathione (in conjunction with vitamin B6, vitamin E and selenium). Note that glutathione is particularly useful at protecting the immune system combating the free radicals which produce an intensification of the aging process, when free radicals interact with protein, resulting in the gradual development of cross links in collagen fibre which is the characteristic sign of aging; detoxifying heavy metals and removing from the body lead, cadmium, mercury and aluminium; the detoxification of liver peroxidation, e.g. alcohol-produced damage of the liver.
- Selenium.
- Essential oils, with the exception of citrus oils which may contain free radicals, unless the fruit is organically grown. (Note that Earl Grey tea can generate free radicals from the oil of bergamot which has three acute carcinogens, whose effects can be exacerbated in the presence of refined sugars, fats, etc.)
- Ionisers are useful for reducing free radical formation, particularly in a car.
- A non-toxic diet (see notes on diet in Chapter 21).
- Detoxifying the body (see notes in Chapter 26).
- Boosting the immune system (see notes in Chapter 8).

Many drugs block the synthesis of DNA and RNA (the genetic material) and are in themselves carcinogenic, damaging normal cells. It is therefore important to boost the immune system and detoxify, both at the same time, to counter the effects of carcinogens so as to inhibit free radical generation, which would otherwise lead to cancer. It is not the cancer cells that need attacking but the free radicals generated by faulty chemical and biochemical processes.

DIET TO STOP FREE RADICAL ACTIVITY

It is essential to separate proteins and carbohydrates when eating, as otherwise there is a quick fermentation, with consequent discomfort. This is the basis of the Hay system of eating (see notes on page 159).

- Meat may be all right in itself but it is mostly now denatured through the use of chemicals so that it has been virtually changed from a biological food to a chemical one.
- Bacteria and fungi (particularly candida) glut on any undigested food and excrete toxins which are potentially carcinogenic. There is bacterial viral or fungal contamination in many foods and the body protests, resulting in bloating.
- A vegetarian diet is no protection as it includes many yeast-infected foods such as mushrooms, dairy products, nuts, pulses, and fruits.
- Barley, rye, wheat, oats are all highly glutenous. Modern hybrid grains have high protein in a different form from the old varieties; they are stickier and more elastic, which the body cannot cope with. Modern oats have a higher level of protein than formerly.
- Rice, corn, millet, buckwheat and bere meal (available in the Orkneys) are all non-glutenous grains, and therefore better. But many cancer patients cannot tolerate even non-glutenous grains because of contamination. Each person is different and it is a question of trial and error to find out if one is allergic or not to a particular grain.
- Note that the longer food remains in the stomach, the more mucus is formed, which may lead to possible infections, ulcerations and free radical change.
- Always cook pulses slowly for a long time, and have vitamin C before pulse meals, to act as an antioxidant to any toxin. It is useful to include kelp or seaweed in the pot while cooking, to 'mop up' free radicals; these can be taken out of the pot after a while if not wanted. Many pulses contain carcinogenic material, in particular red kidney beans, soya beans (all products), broad beans (which one should soak with vitamin C to neutralise compounds which oxidise); the best pulses are mung, lentils, aduki beans, flageolets and chickpeas, and they are better still if they are slightly sprouted (the smaller beans have fewer sulphur compounds in them).
- Good nuts are almonds, hazelnuts, cashews (when not broken), pine kernels, chestnuts, coconuts, apricot kernels. Bad nuts are peeled Brazils, walnuts, pecans (which have been painted and have a high natural level of fungus), pistachios, peanuts.
- Good seeds include pumpkin, sesame, sunflower, linseed. Soak them first in vitamin C, which makes their minerals more available – soak them overnight and they will be all right in the morning. If unsoaked they are always better for a spraying with vitamin C solution. Seeds can be put through the blending machine; they are excellent for breakfast as they are easily available, are easily

digested and have enough enzymes and amino acids as well as a broad range of minerals and vitamins.

- Tropical fruits are good as occasional treats, e.g. pawpaw (papaya), pineapple, kiwi fruit, mango, melon, banana.
- Dried fruit always has fungal residues, therefore wash them well in hot water, or soak them in cold mineral water in vitamin C (say 1 g to ½ pint of water). Hunza apricots are good, as also are dates. Prunes tend to generate wind.
- Never use yeast extracts, which accelerate bacteria production. Useful flavourings are horseradish, mustard, tahini, Vecon (where the yeast is a different kind from normal), miso (has beneficial bacteria), gluten-free soya sauce (such as t'amari).

18
ALLERGIES

We are born with a storehouse of cells in our immune system and, for the most part, with a functionally able thymus gland, and for a number of years we produce more protective cells, all of which are the controllers of our state of health. For instance, if we take in any toxins through respiration, then the cells of the immune system will produce an allergic reaction. Many children are allergic to cow's milk and wheat right from babyhood – a natural response of the body to fend off invasive material. It is important to realise that such babies are not ill; it is a natural response. If Ventolin or hormones are given routinely, then that child's immune responses are undermined and weakened. Many degenerative diseases are iatrogenic (induced by drugs or food) due to the introduction into the body of alien compounds that the body is not designed to handle.

Childhood illnesses are nature's way of eliminating toxic materials from the body. If they are adequately dealt with, perhaps by allowing a fever to run its course and die out, giving only some vitamins, clear soup, etc., while the body shifts a lot of toxins, things will be all right. The object of treatment should be to help the child eliminate its toxins. Do not hinder it and the cleansing process will take place.

Allergies in children also appear as a result of a breakdown in the immune system of the mother, when toxic products pass across the placental barrier into the foetus and perhaps also past its blood/brain barrier. This is happening more and more because the sensorability of the parents' blood barrier is being constantly attacked by a much wider cocktail of trigger factors than in the past, so that a child has little chance of being born 100 per cent healthy.

Prior to a baby's conception, parents should therefore go through a period of detoxification so that at conception the baby will not be the recipient of all the toxic load that cannot be channelled anywhere else once immunity has broken down. Perhaps the mother or father may have been suffering ill health prior to conception. Gradually, as the baby grows, more and more of the mother's toxic load will be diverted to the placenta. She will feel better, but it will only be at the expense of passing on to the foetus toxins which would normally have gone to some of her own organs. If a child inherits this sort of poor 'blueprint', then he is in trouble right from the start.

Most foods children eat are addictive. Foods they eat produce a kind of pre-programming, so if, for instance, they are fed on hormone-impregnated milk, then the child's neurological responses and glandular system will be pre-programmed to accept this type of food. They will act and live in response to what this particular food is doing to them. The child can of course be detoxified later; with the right conditions, such as having a gluten-free diet and not taking a lot of undigestible protein material, the cells will repair themselves and the child's health will improve.

The small intestine is the most permeable organ in the allergic child, so all kinds of toxins get into the bloodstream; the hyperactive child, for example, suffers from a gut that is constantly permeable to toxins, which can pass into the bloodstream and even into the brain itself, through the blood/brain barrier. Their behaviour patterns change quite significantly as a result of this invasion of the brain tissues by toxins.

All degenerative diseases have conditions connected with deep-seated multiple allergies. These begin early in life with a number of allergies that are not attended to; later on, instead of coming to the surface as the symptoms of a response to an invasive organism, they go 'underground', into the deeper tissues affected by the degenerative illness. They must surface again, however, so that one can deal with the original condition that arose in the first place, otherwise one is never able to deal with the roots of the illness.

The body's tissues are constantly irritated by substances that can provoke an allergic response; the body therefore produces extra glandular and mucus secretions to cope with the offending material, with the result that the tissues are then continually inflamed and irritated. Because of this production of extra hormonal secretions and extra white cells to cope with invading material, we introduce into the system a number of hormones and proteins that are not designed to be there in normal processes. They enter the cellular environment and the body has either to get rid of these elements through a strong immune reaction, or allow them to become part of the tissues, even though they do not belong there.

The allergic person is always at risk of developing a malignancy or some sort of illness that causes tissue change, e.g. rheumatoid arthritis, which is a characteristic result of a condition of exacerbation through allergies over a number of years. Gradually there will be very poor assimilation of nutrients, with congestion of the mucous membranes throughout the gastrointestinal tract. Then, gradually, a depletion of essential nutrients occurs and a lot of invasive agents penetrate into the blood and, through the blood, into the joints where the synovial fluid (which is in between the joints) gradually becomes displaced or highly toxic and causes a lot of stress and inflammation in the joints.

DEALING WITH ALLERGIES

The main way to find out what a person is allergic to is through an exclusion diet; all other tests, such as a cytotoxic test, are incomplete. Long-standing allergies to which one may not be showing any reactivity, particularly where the allergy is to a staple food eaten every day, such as gluten in bread, mucoproteins from milk, etc., will not show up in a cytotoxic test; there appears to be a kind of permanent reactivity to the allergic food and the body does not show any alarm responses. If you do without a particular food for a month and then have some, you will notice an immediate allergic response to it – an immediate alarm sounds throughout the body. There may be a lot of mucus production, which is a good sign that the body is responding properly. The allergic mechanism should be welcomed as a mechanism of defence. However, it can become over-exacerbated and produce too many antibodies; if the body becomes over-stimulated in this manner, then it may react to almost everything and will be in a kind of allergic response all the time. An allergy is really a person's protector; it means there is enough immune response to make the allergy obvious.

Another method of finding out what allergens one is suffering from is through an elimination diet. Choose a range of foods that you are not used to, and stick to them for a month, e.g. artichokes, asparagus, chichory, etc. – anything in fact that your body is not used to, including unusual or not-often-eaten meats if you are a meat eater. Choose 20–30 foods that your body is not used to and which are completely different from your normal diet. This is a very good way of learning what your body messages are going to be, after a time, when you have taken away all the possible allergens you have been eating over a long period of time.

There are now disciplines, like clinical ecology and immunology, that have been successful in helping people who would not be helped by orthodox treatment, which operate by excluding offending materials, searching for possible allergens, and then introducing vaccines to enable the individual to eat them regardless of his sensitivity. However, this is a questionable approach as it sends the allergy underground again, allowing the unfolding of degenerative disease in a silent manner; the body will accept this allergic material as being normal, but it will still be doing damage to the tissues. What one should be aiming at is to minimise the reactivity of the body with the positive production of the right antibodies, a much more efficient activation of the immune system and management of one's nutrition so that the body will automatically produce healthy elements for correct cellular order.

Mental confusion is a symptom of allergies, and patients in self-help groups have often helped each other when they were having reactions and suffering from mental confusion as well as depression. Allergies, either obvious or hidden, can make life truly miserable.

19
METABOLIC TYPES

Each of us is unique biochemically and everyone has a different metabolism, these different and biochemical metabolic factors influencing the neurological and glandular characteristics of a person. Metabolic typing is an attempt to define each person's unique genetically determined capacity to convert food into energy. It is useful for anyone with a chronic ailment to recognise what is their basic metabolic type and what are the types of food they should be eating. Indeed many diseases may be the result of cells not receiving the specific nutrients they require, resulting in 'cellular malnutrition' and metabolic dysfunction.

DIFFERENT METHODS OF CATEGORISATION

One system of categorising people with similar emotional, personality and health characteristics is under the two broad headings of sympathetic and parasympathetic types, according to which of the two nervous systems function is the more dominant in the individual, with various grades between the two extremes.

Another system of categorisation uses the following three headings, although in practice it can be seen that people often have some characteristics of two or even all three groupings:

- Endomorphs are soft round people with large digestive organs – slow, amiable and lovers of physical comforts.
- Mesomorphs are heavily built with large bones and muscles – assertive and outgoing.
- Ectomorphs are long and lean – socially inhibited and mentally intense.

They have also been classified as:

- Pituitary – who do well on a vegetarian diet.
- Adrenal – here a high-protein diet is best and they are unable to do well on a vegetarian diet.
- Thyroid types – mixed feeders.

Or people may be thought of more simply as:

- Meat eaters (high-protein eaters), who need 60 per cent of their food to be acid-forming.
- Vegetarians, who may not need any, or only a little, animal protein.
- Mixed feeders, requiring 60–70 per cent of their food to be alkaline.

A simpler version of this last classification is:

- Alkaline types, who do well on animal protein.
- Acid types requiring vegetarian food.
- Balanced types, who seem to thrive on a mixed diet.

This last system of categorising metabolic types has been looked at in some detail by the Nutritional Counselling Service of Dallas, Texas, USA as follows.

TYPE I, HIGHLY ACID TYPES

These people are mostly strongly affected by what is called the 'accelerator', i.e. the sympathetic nervous system. Their acidity activates the influx of calcium and phosphorus into each cell, triggering the brain's nerve transmitters responsible for the sympathetic nervous system.

These are slow metabolisers who utilise sugar at a slow, even, rate and they digest food slowly; therefore they must have easily digested foods. They are very fond of meat, have almost a craving for it, but as meat is difficult to digest and is an acid-forming food (and they are already over-acid) they actually need a mainly vegetarian alkaline diet to balance their acid pH. To be curative their diet should not contain much fat or proteins; fats bind magnesium and prevent efficient calcium utilisation and calcium and phosphorus levels in their cells tend to be high. They usually dislike salty food.

Such people habitually produce too much stomach acid. They are quick, nervous, active people who are enthusiastic but tire easily. There may be a history of repeated infections, tonsillitis, appendicitis, liver problems, glandular fever. They have an over-production of bile and feel nauseated, bring up bile and are easily sick.

They are energetic, thrive on strenuous exercise, are workaholics, leaders, cold and efficient. They have well-proportioned bodies, are tall, with long arms and legs and fingers. The moons on their fingernails are large and well defined. They have strong adrenal glands, and the other endocrine glands are highly developed so they handle stress very well, although if there is no outlet for their stress they may start some form of illness. They may become very intense and anxious and rather reserved. They can tolerate pain well.

Their saliva pH is usually lower than normal (instead of being alkaline as it should be, the saliva will tend towards acidity). The mouth tends to dryness and there is not enough alkaline saliva to start breaking down foods, particularly the mucopolysaccharides such as gluten, with the result that the stomach is unable to break the food down much further, creating further problems for the small intestines where the main carbohydrate digestion takes place.

They commonly have strong mood swings. They do not bottle up their feelings so can release and express their feelings and therefore are more able to deal with their emotional life. There are probably more possibilities for real healing in a highly acidic individual.

They eat quickly and do not gain weight. There is much flatulence and wind if they eat certain vegetables. As children they strongly dislike vegetables and salads. They may be hyperactive. As babies they show their type clearly, even at birth.

They are looser in their motions, and have wind from the waist down (alleviated by homoeopathic lycopodeum).

In the stomach pepsin and rennin act on ingested protein. If however the saliva is too acid it would not start the breaking down process as there would not have been enough bicarbonate to neutralise the acid, so food that is not broken down properly enters the duodenum, together with acid chyme (the semi-liquid mixture of partly digested foods and acid from the stomach) and this counteracts the effect of the alkaline pancreas enzyme secretions which would not then be able to break down the starches and sugars adequately.

Acid types are always over-producing mucus (mucoproteins) and therefore continuously transporting undigested particles of food through the gut into the blood. Suppose one eats toast and marmalade. This consists of a plant hormone and protein (from the wheat in the toast) plus an animal protein and hormone (from butter) plus activator or fermenting agent. The sugars and fats which are emulsified become tightly locked to each other by the mucus and can pass into the blood unchecked and undigested. These particles can then help form tumours, or lodge in the weakest parts such as the joints producing arthritis, or gradually thicken the blood, making it sluggish and resulting in toxins accumulating in the lymph glands.

Type I metabolisers do have good calcium metabolism, resulting in adequate to excess calcium.

Diseases to which this type are very prone include bacterial infections, diabetes, ulcerative colitis, rheumatoid arthritis, arteriosclerosis, cancer, high blood pressure, heartburn, heart arrhythmias.

Some characteristics of this type are as follows:

- Often constipated but regular every two or three days.
- Get to sleep easily, but often insomnia later.
- Normal appetite, but 'picky'.
- Rely on stimulants to keep going.
- Idealistic, creative.
- Strong sexual desires.
- Tolerate pain well.
- Prone to headaches.
- Dislike salty food.
- Have periods of activity, interspersed with inactivity.
- Have a tendency to catch infections.

Vitamins and minerals that are particularly required by this group include vitamins B1, B2, B6, PABA, niacin, vitamins C and D, potassium, magnesium, copper, manganese and ferrous sulphate. Note that L-tyrosine or L-dopa are precursors of noradrenaline, which increases the metabolic rate and has a thermogenic (i.e. fat-burning) and appetite-suppressing effect.

TYPE II, HIGHLY ALKALINE TYPES

These people are at the other end of the scale. They are most strongly affected by their weaker parasympathetic nervous system or 'decelerator', with greater nerve stimulation, through the vagus and pelvic nerves, to the gastrointestinal tract.

They are generally fast metabolisers and, through having a highly developed pancreas, they are fast sugar oxidisers who may develop hypoglycaemia. They digest food quickly but eat too much. They should not be encouraged to become vegetarians as fruit and leafy vegetables, being high in potassium, lower calcium levels (which are lower than normal in these types anyhow). They produce excess histamine (partly due to a deficiency in calcium levels) and adrenaline production is lower than normal (adrenaline is an anti-histamine). They need slow-burning acid-forming foods like healthy meat and fats (fats help to slow down the oxidation rate). Dairy products provide high levels of calcium and fat so are good for these types on both counts. They are liable to put on weight easily and become overweight.

They produce very little stomach acid, and therefore thrive on a high animal protein diet of meat and other acid-forming foods, especially fatty high-purine meats like red meat, salmon, tuna, dairy products, butter, oils, while they should restrict the amounts of bread, grains, cereals and fruit. They are often constipated and often tend towards obesity. In the stomach the limited hydrochloric acid secretion means that pepsin (a protein-digesting enzyme) is not activated and digestion of any proteins is delayed and inadequate.

Continuous regurgitation of food is a feature of alkaline types. Similarly, wind in the upper part of the body denotes an alkaline type (for which homoeopathic carbo. veg. is helpful).

They are less active and slower than acid types, and often can become introverted and pessimistic. Their medical history shows very little physical illness, but they can become neurotic and hypochondriacal.

They often have osteoarthritis, and fibroids. There are problems of calcification and retention of alkaline elements in the bloodstream, as well as in the joints; this gives rise to problems such as MS and osteoarthritis, both of which are related to high alkalinity.

There may be liver problems, as liver function is better in acid types. This may mean tumour growth, fibroids (fibroids in an organ means the person involved is probably an alkaline type) or cirrhosis of the liver, particularly if the individual is an alcoholic. Brandy, whisky, vodka – in fact any of the distillates – will probably result in cirrhosis of the liver. Through drinking large quantities of fermented drinks such as beer, wine or soft drinks, there is likely to be liver cancer or hepatitis B, because the drinks produce ferments that in turn encourage lots of yeast organisms in the liver to proliferate.

They have poorly developed endocrine systems.

Diseases to which this type are very prone include asthma, low blood pressure, hypoglycaemia, diverticulitis, oedema, hayfever, viral infections, mucous colitis.

Characteristics of this type are as follows:

- Cravings for salty foods; prefer proteins.
- Can eat anything; strong digestion, with frequent bowel movements.
- Hands and feet normally warm.
- Flabby under-developed muscles.
- Quick-clotting blood; low blood pressure.
- Slow to anger; easy going, gregarious, sociable, outgoing.
- Make decisions after careful thought.
- Not easily aroused sexually.
- Have strong teeth, short fingers, stocky build, good facial colour.
- Tend to put on weight easily.

- Sensitive to effects of even small stresses, which can lead to health problems; prone to depressions.
- Strong resistance to infections; strong immune system.
- Slow starters in the morning.

Vitamins and minerals that are particularly required include vitamins A, B12, B3, B5 (important), B6, choline, inositol, vitamin E, bioflavinoids, garlic, calcium, phosphorus, iodine, zinc, selenium. These types should not have food high in potassium, such as molasses, alfalfa, bananas (which are too alkaline), nor much in the way of grains due to their high phytic acid content which tends to lower calcium levels (these types already show a calcium deficiency).

TYPE III, BALANCED TYPES

This group consists of individuals who are flexible and fall halfway between types I and II. They have a urine pH of about 5.9.
    Some characteristics of this type include:

- Delicate build; thin, long neck; silky fine hair.
- Easily aroused nervous system.
- More likely to be fast metabolisers.
- Easily dissatisfied; easily fatigued.
- Lack concentration; some insomnia.
- Mixed feeders; best on low-salt diet.
- Need calcium-rich foods, including dairy products.

The diet should exclude salt and cut down on red meat, sugar, refined flour or rice. It should include dairy products, yoghourt, etc. Supplements should include the B vitamins, selenium, zinc, kelp and dolomite (for calcium and magnesium).

METABOLIC TYPE AND DIET

As can be seen, each type requires specific kinds of diet supplementation, with very specific vitamins, minerals and other nutrients.
    One's original 'blueprint' is for a balanced individual, and healthy people can change from being acidic to being alkaline, or vice versa, quite easily. If, however, a person is particularly one or the other there is a danger of imminent degenerative disease. People become ill because they have gone one way or another, i.e. they have become acid or alkali against their basic nature. This may have happened because of some shock or trauma; for instance if a child is sent to a boarding school

at seven, thereby moving from a liberal environment to a much more restraining and disciplinarian regime, he or she will suffer a sudden shock which can convert them from an acid type to an alkaline type very easily. These swings from acidity to alkalinity can be seen in the medical history and will often correspond with the traumatic changes in their lives.

If a child inherits a poor metabolic blueprint, then they are in trouble right from the start. If a child very early on shows signs of hyperactivity and acidity it will not be long before they show degenerative illness. Equally, if the mother was ill during pregnancy this will affect her baby, although this trend can be reversed if dealt with in good time.

It can therefore be seen that our capacity to use the food we eat and transform the nutrients in it depends entirely on our whole organism. We can consciously change our way of living today and see that our children do not suffer similarly. As adults we may now be having to cope with disease because of a long history of suppression, or shock, or repeated alterations of metabolic type whereby we have rarely had a metabolic balance all our lives – we become ill because we swing from one condition to the other, in response to whatever is thrust on us in the way of social conditioning, family pressures, dieting, work and emotional stress.

The acidity or alkalinity of a person ties up not only with the diet, but also with the shocks and traumas which affect the digestive organs. As these organs have the task of providing the blood with nutrients extracted from food taken into the body, any disturbance of their working will result in the body not getting sufficient nourishment, and disease will follow. Incompletely broken-down substances will further disturb pH balance and will enter the bloodstream and then go to various organs and disturb their function. Bacterial action in the intestines, fuelled by the wrong foods and an unbalanced pH, can then introduce toxins into the bloodstream. Our endocrine glands are all the while trying to compensate, so that despite emotional and other stresses, most people manage to reach a balance.

TESTS TO DETERMINE METABOLIC CATEGORY

Tests that you can do for yourself to determine what category you fit into have been suggested as follows:

- Take 50 mg of niacin (vitamin B3) on an empty stomach. If, within 30 minutes, you feel hot and itchy and your skin appears reddened, you fall into the meat-eating group. If you feel just slightly warmer and your face colours a little, you are a balanced type. If nothing happens, you are a natural vegetarian.

- Take 8 grams of ascorbic acid (vitamin C) each day for three days. If you feel lethargic, tired and depressed (with vaginal irritation in women) you should increase your protein intake, especially meat, fish and other proteins and fats. The balanced type will feel no change. The natural vegetarian will feel better than usual, sleep well and have more energy.

20
ELECTROMAGNETIC FORCES AND THE BIOPHYSICAL SHIELD

ELECTROMAGNETIC FORCES

The electromagnetic forces of a person are normally very strong, but when people are continuously submitted to very poor nutrition and therefore their food intake contains very little in the way of electromagnetically charged minerals and metals, then their magnetic fields get very weak. Scanners to detect the electromagnetic fields of the individual can tell where the resonance of a person is going wrong; they can easily identify, in pictures, where the electromagnetic conductivity of the cells is poor or does not exist.

If a person's electromagnetism is low, they will be subject to electromagnetic radiation from outside the body, i.e. interference from the environment interpenetrating cellular material. An NMR machine at Surrey University, capable of showing up blood trace elements, can pick up differences in the electromagnetic metals, particularly cobalt, manganese and magnesium in the body, and also the changes that come into the blood and body fluids when people live directly underneath overhead power cables. A survey in the Ferndown area of Dorset, comprising just over 1,000 people living near or under overhead cables, showed that of those 1,000 people 144 developed cancers, made up of 53 childhood cancers (including 25 leukaemias, 20 of whom lived near hydrant valves) while the adults contracted leukaemia (22), brain tumours (17), lung cancer (6), lymphomas (4), cancer of the uterus (4), breast cancer (8), cancers of the skin (3), spine (3), stomach (8), bowel (3), liver (2), throat and oesophagus (2), kidney and bladder (2), pancreas (2), testicles (2), ovary (1), jaw (1) and a myleoma (1).

It must be said that the effect of the overhead power lines may not be the only, or even the main, cause of these cancers, although statistically the figures are very significant. It does become more important, though, if the person's nutritional, and in particular their mineral, status is poor. And it shows the effect that external radiation can have on the electromagnetic field of the individual and, through it, the person's cellular health.

Microwaves change the electromagnetism of the food. As we are concerned with our own electrical conductivity, which is altered during any degenerative illness, it is a sensible precaution to use microwaves only minimally, for heating rather than for cooking (although to date there is no substantial scientific evidence of any adverse effects being obtained from the use of microwave cookers).

THE BIOPHYSICAL SHIELD

All our organs have their own electromagnetic fields which interact with the earth's field, with other energy fields and with the energy fields of other people nearby – encephalographs (EEGs) can measure our brain waves, ECGs record energy waves from the heart, EMGs from muscles. Similarly, energy fields extend beyond the surface of the body and can be detected 12 to 15 inches from the surface of the body by a 'sensitive' person. This is because every cell in the body has got an electrical charge, and all the cells build up a 'bio-magnetic' field round the body, as shown by NMR scanners; these clearly show that the energy field round a person is quite large, larger than the person, and acts as a shield against any other magnetised particles that are trying to enter that space.

This field, being larger than the person, will tend to overlap the field of anyone sitting close by, and therefore one person's field can be felt by someone else a short distance away. Most of us are not aware of this in our daily lives, but if one thinks lovingly of one's neighbour, then he or she will feel that expression of love or warmth. This energy field, or aura, has been well known in the east for centuries and medicine men in all kinds of cultures have been able to heal by the reconstitution of the 'auric body'. This is basically what a healer is doing to a patient, although often unconsciously.

If the protective shield is healthy, then the body processes do not break down, cells regenerate normally, oxygen is converted to carbon dioxide, blood and lymph move, muscle development takes place, etc. But if the energy body gets damaged, then a lot of alterations take place in the physical body. When we become ill, any cells that have broken down (or altered their magnetic resonance) will therefore be discernible through the use of an NMR scanner; thus the nature of the 'biofield' of the individual can be revealed, allowing us to measure and assess where the cells have broken down or where they have altered their magnetic status. This protective shield actually physically lessens the response of our glands and nerves to outside trauma, whether physical or mental.

The situation can be reversed though. Perhaps you are faced with a most horrid problem, but you find that you have the presence of mind to step outside the situation so that you are untouched, unaffected by it, thus minimising the impact the emotional turmoil might have had on a stable physiology. However, if you were overwhelmed by the problem you would find that you were in a state approaching that of permanent shock; your pituitary, thyroid and adrenal glands would be constantly overstimulated, so that the hormones produced by these glands are raised dramatically to abnormal levels. At these levels the hormones and their breakdown products can be harmful and have a deleterious effect on the biophysical electromagnetic field that surrounds us. With this shield compromised, we are then prey to more damage from electromagnetic or low-ionising radiation attacks.

Life today is not only afflicting us with a remorseless stream of stresses and shocks. We are ourselves also liable to relive and dwell on these stresses and shocks, going over and over them, either consciously or subconsciously. And each time we do this we trigger some physiological reactions. The result can be an almost permanent assault on our biophysical shield, from within. It is therefore important that we not only learn to cope with these stresses but that we also learn to exorcise the memories of them.

21
FOOD

SPEED OF DIGESTION – OUR 'METABOLIC' CLOCK

Proteins are digested in 3½ to 4 hours, provided they have not been denatured by cooking. If they are, and all the enzymes within the food have been destroyed, it will take 7–10 hours, according to how tough the protein is – tough protein will linger on in the stomach where it gradually putrefies. Some people have undigested protein lying in the stomach for up to 36 hours. How does this situation arise?

It is quite common to have a large meal and then have a cup of coffee with sugar. It takes 1½ hours to break down simple carbohydrates (such as potatoes without their skins), 4 hours approximately to break down proteins and complex carbohydrates, and 7–10 hours to break down denatured proteins. What happens is that the digestive clock is 'set' to the denominator, the food element, which is the fastest absorbed into the blood, i.e. the sugar. If we set the digestive clock at the end of a meal to the processing of sugars rather than proteins, then all the digestive functions are geared to clear the sugars, not the proteins and not the complex carbohydrates. The simple sugars are therefore digested and absorbed but proteins and complex carbohydrates stay there undigested until the next meal comes along.

Complex carbohydrates (such as whole grains, or potatoes in their jackets, which have a lot of cellulose interlinked with the sugars and starches in their skins) take between 3½–4 hours too, so, as long as the protein is partially predigested, e.g. by soaking in a marinade, etc., then it and the carbohydrates will both pass into the gut together and the bacteria there will be able to cope with the components of both the partially digested protein and the carbohydrates at the same time. They can therefore be mixed together, providing the items of food all go through the stomach into the gut at the same time harmoniously (i.e. their digestive clocks are synchronised).

Potatoes without their skins are simple carbohydrates. Rice with fish or seafoods is acceptable, but rice with lamb is much heavier. Roast meat with potatoes, Yorkshire pudding, etc., sets the metabolic clock to the simple carbohydrates in the Yorkshire pudding and potatoes, and not to the meat, which therefore will not get properly digested when eaten together.

FOOD DURING ILL HEALTH

In the olden days people ate few, or very few, varieties of food and were still moderately healthy. In poor countries there are still people who have not had more than a handful of different foods all their lives, and yet they are healthy and live very long useful lives well into their 80s and 90s. It is not therefore a question of variety of food, but of quality that affects us. Perhaps the human organism is really designed to cope with only a few foods at a time. Today there is a very large variety of foods, even at one meal – perhaps 30 or more different substances at one sitting, many of which may, chemically or biochemically, be fighting each other inside us, the consequences being cell damage.

The idea of a diet brings up the spectre of restrictions in most people's minds, and this in itself can cause unnecessary stress. But, diets for people who are ill are very personal things. What suits one person will not suit another, so experimentation is required with foods that are beneficial rather than harmful. It all depends on a person's metabolism. If the body is metabolising too fast and having difficulty in absorbing protein, it is better to have the protein meal early in the day. Proteins put the body into a catabolic state (a breaking-down process), whereas carbohydrates are much more involved in building up (the anabolic process). It is therefore worth considering changing meals around and having a protein meal at midday instead of in the evening, or vice versa.

Cancer patients are very similar to coeliacs – indeed they may have been coeliacs without being diagnosed as such. There may have been ulcers in the gut and, as time goes by, the gut becomes coated with a thick layer of mucus and the wrong kind of bacteria. To change this condition, and get the gut functioning again so that it can absorb nutrients, we must have easily absorbable food with a broad spectrum of nutrients, such as juices, predigested nuts and pulses and sprouted seeds (just sprouted, at the stage where they are just beginning to show a little shoot). Pumpkin, sesame and sunflower seeds all contain coenzyme Q_{10}, which is absolutely essential in the metabolism of cells. Nature always provides the necessary nutrients and it is only now that industry is finding out what is required.

As cancer is a mental starvation as well as a physical one, it is essential to make foods look interesting. A diet of juice alone requires enormous dedication and is likely to fail. To make life interesting, have 'rainbow' meals with a spectrum of foods with different colours, resulting in a meal with variety; for instance, what about an entrée of avocado with prawns, or with sauce of lemon juice, olive oil, garlic and grain mustard on a bed of colourful salad?

If you are having digestive problems when you are ill, think of yourself as a baby and give your body food accordingly. You are then giving yourself a chance to allow formative and restorative activity again. This is particularly necessary if someone has a sensitive gut with digestive disturbances and inflammations, in which case it is important to reduce the amount of inflammation, ulcerated tissues, etc., which need to be healed.

When we are ill and have difficulty in assimilating nutrients it is important to eat only food that is easily absorbed. There is a lot of nutrition in seeds or nuts, but they are very hard to eat if you are not feeling well. It is better to wash them, soak them (thereby 'predigesting' them, making them more tender and releasing enzymes), liquidise them and incorporate them in soup, a dip, or a spread for a biscuit, which then makes a very good attractive and nutritious food.

If the gut is contaminated by the wrong types of organisms, i.e. the anaerobic organisms, then in order to survive they are profiting from our own nutrients and blood, rather than working for us as the aerobic organisms do, which demolish the food and transport nutrients so that we can make healthy blood, build up tissues, etc. Good bacteria in the gut are those that use oxygen to help us digest our food and make it possible for us to take in nutrients rather than toxins from the food. However, if there are colicky pains, distension, burning, a wheezy feeling in the intestinal tract, this all means we are probably colonised by anaerobic organisms (which work without oxygen and produce harmful chemicals); we therefore come to need supplements to keep us going so that our health will be maintained as we will not be profiting from the food we have eaten. Furthermore, these unpleasant symptoms are always indicative of a high level of mucus build-up along the intestinal tract, from the oesophagus downwards.

It may be thought that yeasts are destroyed by cooking at a high temperature. This is true, but the mycotoxins that they produce are not destroyed. And some yeasts, primarily the 'bad' ones such as *Candida albicans*, have to be heated to a very high temperature to kill them. So if we cook food we therefore destroy most proteins and nutrients, and if we do not cook the food we get contaminated by fungi, bacteria and viruses. The only safe method is to soak and marinade proteins, particularly all meats, nuts and seeds. In this way we release the enzymes in the food and allow them to destroy microorganisms effectively.

It is important for nerve function and the glands to extract minerals from food, and this is a justification for cooking some foods, as it helps release the minerals and metals. There is no great value in cooked food from the point of view of amino acids, enzymes or vitamins, but there is from the aspect of the minerals and fibre. Most fats become toxic after cooking, especially when the liver, gallbladder and/or pancreas fail to deliver pancreatic enzymes and biles, because there are then no enzymes left in the food to help digest them. Here avocados are useful as they have fats, with enzymes, that don't need cooking. It is better to steam or quickly sauté vegetables, as in a wok, so that the vegetables release their minerals quickly; in this way the individual can generate a lot of neurological energy, (nerve energy) which is dependent on mineral and metal availability. It is therefore good not to eat all food raw but to have some foods slowly steamed or stir-fried.

The most important thing when you change your lifestyle and way of eating is to understand why you are doing it, so that you know, if you transgress, how to correct it. If you know a certain food is going to disturb you, blow you up, etc., take vitamin C before and after having the food to prepare the tissues, so that the cells will not be so badly damaged or inflamed. It is quite useful to take vitamin C in vegetable juices. However, don't take a lot of offending foods, thinking that the vitamin C will counteract any bad effects. It is all right occasionally to give yourself a treat, but protect yourself from the consequences.

SUNDRY POINTS

- In any degenerative disease one should use as many foods as possible that are predigested so that the body has the minimum of work to do to break them down into the components required by the blood; otherwise the body will be carrying toxicity and material that is not adequately broken down, a lot of which will remain in the gut or will be laid down as very long-chain saturated fatty acids or complex microproteins somewhere in the tissues.
- When considering what to eat it is useful to consider eating as many small meals (about five or six a day) as possible rather than having a huge meal once a day.
- Digestion should begin in the mouth, where the mechanical action of the jaws plus the alkaline salivary juices start the breakdown of all food.
- Do not drink with meals, but drink at least eight glasses of water or juice a day, sipping small amounts. Ideally the water should be good bottled mineral water or water that has been treated through a reverse osmosis system.
- A lot of vegetarian food is highly suspect, much of it being highly contaminated, particularly with yeast.

- Wholemeal bread is more toxic than white bread unless the grain is adequately treated. Even organically grown grain is still affected by environmental toxins and mould, which is a pity as wholemeal bread is so much more nourishing.
- All vegetables should be raw or gently steamed or sautéed – never overcooked. They can be flavoured with such things as kelp powder, seasalt, plain Korean pepper, raw or unsalted butter (not pasteurised), olive, sesame or linseed oils.
- Always start a meal with something raw, i.e. something that has not been degraded; this will set the metabolic clock off correctly so that the subsequent digestive activity is regulated by the acids and enzymes that have been produced when eating the raw food.
- Microwaves are useful for defrosting foods, but if you cook with them you quickly destroy any enzymes in the food. It is, however, possible to arrange the microwave to cook very slowly so that there is no oscillation of the molecules in the food and the enzymes are preserved but beware when using meats, eggs, fish, or convenience foods. If you use the microwave only to defrost you are not heating the food for long enough to destroy the enzymes within it.
- Anything hot in the morning tends to cause mucus; therefore it is better to have something like yoghourt first thing, before a cup of tea.
- Anything with fungus on it should not be eaten. Fungus can produce a substantial bacterial colony within a couple of hours, one organism producing millions.
- If there is mould, say, on top of some jam, most people will remove it and then eat the jam. But the chemicals those microorganisms have produced (i.e. the mycotoxins) have not been removed and can do as much damage as the mould itself.
- Always wash very well all nuts, seeds, pulses, etc., or soak them overnight or until they are just sprouting, then dry them, e.g. by putting them in a microwave for a short time. Most nuts and seeds are contaminated with yeasts, so wash them in vitamin C to neutralise the toxins.
- It is useful to spend a bit of time preparing something to have the next day, when you might want a snack and may not feel like preparing a meal. One suggestion is to mix miso and tahini, sesame seeds, garlic, chives or parsley. This makes a nice spread. Inside tortillas you can put many things such as avocados, cucumbers, vegetable stew, grated carrots, etc.
- Any damaged vegetables can be carcinogenic. Vegetables, wherever they are cut or damaged, produce chemicals (psoralens) to limit the

risk of further damage from invading bacteria and fungi, and psoralens are carcinogenic. Similarly, grains produce chemicals in their fight against fungi. Such chemicals are also formed as soon as fruit or vegetables start to oxidise; therefore spray vegetables with vitamin C or put into them antioxidants such as vitamin C, garlic or onions. Note that psoralens are potent light-activated carcinogens and mutagens widespread in plants of the umbelliferae family such as celery, parsley and figs. They increase enormously when the plants are under unusual stress such as sudden changes in temperatures or when being 'force-fed' with high levels of fertilisers. They damage DNA molecules and produce oxygen radicals in the presence of sunlight or fluorescent light.

- What is a typical diet for a week? This is up to the individual to construct a programme based on non-glutenous food that he or she likes most – but without sugar. This is a matter for thought, not worry. Have fun in preparing suitable foods. Take recipes from any recipe book and adapt them if necessary to take into account the special requirements of your body.

A SHOPPING BASKET

The Springhill basic food programme is, in general, common to all participants at the Centre, whatever health problem is involved. It is one which an increasing number of people, without apparent health problems, are seeking as a means of working towards preventative health care.

The back-to-health process is one which starts with acknowledging the problem, and then taking positive steps which might include a combination of healthy practices, such as relaxation exercises, seeking a cleaner environment, as well as healthy food.

If the food programme selected contains tasty, satisfying, attractive meals which are relatively simple to prepare, then there will be a greater inclination to follow the Springhill nutritional guidelines. Emphasis is placed upon those foodstuffs which are in harmony with the basic principles already mentioned. A positive response by the participant will do much to aid a more relaxed approach and is helpful in encouraging a spirit of exploration and discovery.

The nutrition sessions at Springhill include the development of a greater awareness of the individual's unique response to different foods and to varying combinations of food. Methods of production or processing can of course result in changes for good, or ill. The foods that follow are those available in 1990 which can be selected and enjoyed, and, hopefully, whose production and processing will not be tampered with in the foreseeable future.

- Aids to digestion and elimination – linseed (golden variety if possible); oat germ/bran; psyllium husks.
- Beverages – dandelion root coffee; a variety of herb teas such as rosehip, camomile, mango, fennel; vegetable juices freshly extracted, good quality mineral water, coconut milk, kefir.
- Bread substitutes – corn tortillas; gluten-free bread; sprouted grain bread; home-made, not yeast-leavened, muffins, drop scones, pancakes; poppadums, rice cakes, crackers.
- Cereals/grains/flours (organically produced if possible; use whole grains whenever possible, and coarsely milled rather than finely milled flours) – buckwheat flour or whole, roasted or unroasted; cornflakes, sugar-free if possible and vacuum-packed to avoid rancidity; corn, maize, potato and rice flours; whole brown, wild or puffed rice; tortillas, pearl barley; quinoa, tapioca, sage.
- Canned foods – anchovies, artichoke hearts, asparagus, chestnut (whole or purée), cod roe (without preservatives), corn in water (without sugar), herrings, octopus, olives, pilchards, palm hearts, sardines, tomatoes (whole, chopped or puréed), water chestnuts; no salmon.
- Fats – butter (raw or unsalted, preferably Dutch); cheese (goats' or ewes' in moderation); ghee; goats' or ewes' milk (avoid all pasteurised products, which include all commercial yoghourts, even those described as 'live'); piima yoghourt, available from Springhill, but not on mail order; goats' milk with acidophilus.
- Fruits – avocado, apples (cooked), cantaloupe melon, grapefruit, (pink), kiwi fruit, lemons (use for marinading and in salad dressings).
- Nuts and seeds – almonds, cashews, hazelnuts, coconut, linseed, pumpkin seeds (wash and soak in vitamin C solution overnight before use), sesame seeds, sunflower seeds.
- Oils – grapeseed, linseed, olive, sesame, all cold-pressed; avoid all heat-treated oils, including corn and safflower.
- Fish – deep sea varieties (avoid all shallow water fish) such as cod, haddock, herring, hake, halibut, mullet (red), octopus, salmon (wild, not farmed), scallops, shark, swordfish, squid, turbot.
- Meats – if you are not vegetarian, select meats which are from animals raised naturally, without growth hormones and antibiotics, and pasture-fed without mixed grains; game, hare, pigeon, partridge, pheasant, wild rabbit; venison; lamb, all cuts; maize-fed chicken; wild boar; Parma ham.

- Dried vegetables – wash all pulses and soak well overnight in a weak vitamin C solution; beans (use sprouted whenever possible) such as butter, haricot, kidney, lima, mung; chick peas, lentils, peas.
- Fresh vegetables – preferably organically grown, use in large quantities, e.g. artichokes, globe or Jerusalem, asparagus, aubergine, beans, beetroot, broccoli, cabbage, calabrese, cauliflower, celeriac, celery (not bruised and use in season only), chinese leaf, courgettes, corn (whole or as kernels), fennel, kohl rabi, leeks, marrow, okra, onions, parsnips (avoid brown bruised parts), peas, potatoes (avoid all but organically grown and cut away any green tinged potatoes), radish, salad vegetables (chicory, chives, lettuce, cress, sorrel, purslane), shallots, spinach, swede, swiss chard, tomatoes (only freshly gathered or tinned); turnip, watercress, yams.
- Frozen vegetables – green beans, broad beans only infrequently, broccoli, corn, peas, swedes, carrots (without added sugar).
- Seasonings/condiments/flavourings – cayenne pepper (avoid white/black peppercorns), carob powder, cumin, curry spices, garlic (use frequently), ginger (dried or fresh); fresh herbs whenever possible, olives (if in brine rinse and then cover with cold pressed oil), paprika, raising agent (gluten-free), salt (potassium and herb, but with only low sodium), sesame paste such as tahini; spices such as caraway, chilli, cinnamon, coriander, cloves, garam masala, ginger, mace, oregano, paprika, poppy seeds, saffron, turmeric.
- Water – filtered, used for soaking nuts and seeds and for cooking purposes; spring water for drinking (Scottish Spring, Volvic and Spa are recommended as their analysis is satisfactory).

FOODS AND DRINKS TO BE AVOIDED

- Alcohol – beers, lagers, wines; an occasional distilled alcoholic drink is acceptable.
- Butter, salted and pasteurised.
- Black and white peppercorns.
- Cheese (cows'), including cottage-type and blue/green veined cheeses.
- Damaged or mouldy fruit and vegetables.
- Dried fruit.
- Farmed fish such as trout, salmon, oysters.
- Fermented foods – vinegars, soya products such as tofu, pickles, Marmite, Oxo, yeast extract products.

- Fruit produced with pesticides and fungicides, or irradiated.
- Fruit juices, commercially produced especially in aluminium cartons.
- Glutenous grains, oats, rye and barley and products made from them.
- Margarines in general.
- Meats produced with hormones or antibiotics or grains, such as beef, pork, chicken and farmed game.
- Cows' milk.
- Mushrooms (commercial varieties with suspect toxins).
- Oils which have been heat-treated.
- Peanuts and peanut butter.
- Rancid and roasted nuts – shelled walnuts and brazils are prone to rancidity.
- Smoked and pickled fish, meat, poultry, bacon, ham.
- Sugar in all forms, e.g. honey, sweets, preserves (even sugar-free varieties).
- Vegetables raised with inorganic fertilisers and pesticides; limp or bruised vegetables; if in doubt wash and soak briefly in vitamin C solution.
- Wheat products – bread made from wheat; biscuits; cakes; pastries; all products made with wheat flour.
- Yeast – in beer, bread, vegetable extracts, bouillon powders and cubes; dietary supplements unless guaranteed yeast-free.

22

AN ABC OF FOODS

APPLES

Cooked dessert apples do not need added sugar, as cooking apples do sometimes. Raw apples are high in salicylates and encourage fungal growth, but if they are stewed, without sugar, they are quite suitable. They contain magnesium, sulphur, silicon, bromine and vitamins A and C. Baked apples are better than raw, but you lose enzymes and vitamins by baking them, so only have them for the taste rather than for their food value.

Apple juice in cartons encourages a rapid fungal growth. Yeast colonises very quickly on any juices or fermented alcohol, or any yeast foods.

AVOCADOS

Avocados are very easy to digest, and are a delightful base for such entrées as large prawns or scollops, with a marinade of lemon juice, mustard, chopped parsley, olive oil. A sandwich of avocado and tomato is delicious. They can be eaten either with a carbohydrate meal, or be combined with a protein meal as they aid protein digestion. They blend well with all cooked or raw vegetables and with exotic fruits. Make sure that the avocado is not too soft, as in this case the oils can be rancid. If only half is to be eaten at any one time the other half should be covered with vitamin C or lemon juice to stop it from discolouring, a sign of oxidation. It stays in the stomach for a maximum of an hour.

BANANAS

The central part of the banana is often infiltrated by fungi and that is why it tends to go mouldy inside. Bananas can be fried or put in a microwave with a little butter, as a treat. Raw bananas always cause fermentation because of their high sugar content. If, however, they suit you, then it is all right to have them. They take between 45 minutes and two hours to pass through the stomach, which is a longer time than other juicy fruits. Bananas release energy, and, because of this, professional tennis players can often be seen having one between games; if you are hungry between meals, a banana will help to satisfy your hunger. Eat it well away from other meals.

Bananas are alkaline, and low in calories (about 85–90 per banana). They contain three essential amino acids, about one-fifth of the daily requirement of vitamin C, a quantity of vitamin A and some vitamin B and B6. They also have calcium, phosphorus, iron, potassium, magnesium, chlorine and a trace of bromine. They have pectin, which helps digestion. They also help with water retention problems of the kidneys, and can help lead to loss of weight in some cases.

BARLEY

Soak barley for two days. Barley water is a good diuretic and is full of enzymes. Note: it is best to wash the barley (and similarly rice) very well before soaking it.

BEANS

Beans are carbohydrates when they are unsprouted. If, however, they are sprouted they become mostly predigested proteins, so wash any beans or pulses well and sprout for two days. If they are merely soaked overnight, the starches will not have been processed to become protein, vitamins and enzymes, in which case there would be a clash of protein and starches, which makes for a lot of discomfort and sulphorous gases will form. They can be used raw or in any cooking, e.g. in lentil loaf, burgers, rissoles, or liquidised if preferred and used in soups.

Any pulses are highly indigestible for most cancer patients, or anyone who has a condition where the tissues are undergoing change, as in the other degenerative diseases. We always need grains to be predigested when we are ill as the first thing to give way in a degenerative disease process will be the digestive system.

BEETROOT

Beetroot contain flavonoids, which are good for cell respiration, detoxification processes and for countering irradiation or X-ray damage. They are also good for tumours and leukaemia, and give resistance to colds if taken (as juice from two beetroots) daily. They can, however, cause flatulence in some instances. Sometimes they contain a high level of nitrates. If cooked for a short time the nitrates are converted to nitrites, the lesson being to cook them well, simmering for a couple of hours.

BUTTER

Unsalted butter is acceptable. It is preserved in lactic acid and is much more digestible. It is unpasteurised. Butter is the only cows' product which retains the butyric acid, in an easily absorbable form to help in cell repair.

With skimmed milk, full cream cows' milk or cheeses or yoghourts, you are taking in a lot of proteins and compounds, including nitrates that the animal takes in from the cereals it is fed on. Butter has been skimmed, leaving only the fat molecules containing the butyric acid, so as long as butter is pure and natural it is acceptable. Eskimos who live on a very oily diet never got coronaries before they started eating glutenous foods, but the sticky stuff that comes from grains envelops butter or oil particles and makes a gluey material that sticks against the walls of veins and arteries of the lymphatic canals causing tissue changes and degeneration.

CARROTS

Carrot juice has a very high level of sugar. Because of this, carrots increase the candidiasis problem, although the sugar is not released immediately. Raw carrots can be eaten on their own or in salads.

Carrot juice (very high in sugar) has long been used as part of a cancer diet due to its beta-carotene. It is better to use it in combination with other juices (perhaps cabbage, lettuce, celery, dandelion leaves, raspberry leaves, etc.), all juiced together so that the pH of the juices is brought back to equilibrium, with the result that the sugar is not released so fast into the blood and the candidiasis problem does not arise. If it is difficult to have carrot juice mixed with the other vegetables, have a 'tipple' of green vegetables liquidised first, then have the carrot juice with some vitamin C.

CELERY

Celery tea helps to remove excess uric acid and is therefore good for gout, arthritis, rheumatism, lumbago and neuralgia. Put 2 tablespoons of celery seeds in 2 quarts of water and simmer for 3 hours. Strain. Take a cupful three or four times a day, hot, plus celery to eat.

Celery has organic sodium, which helps to keep inorganic sodium in solution so that some of it can be eliminated.

CHEESE

The only cheeses that are safe for most patients to take are very mild cheeses like goats' cheeses, or feta cheese which is a simple curd, never pasteurised, made from sheep's milk, but check that the feta in the shop is not made from cows' milk as it is sometimes, and that it is made from herds which are tested for listeria and other pathogens.

The level of fungus in blue-veined cheeses is quite high.

COCONUT

Have a piece of coconut when you feel the need to have something sweet. Roughcut coconut is useful, or get a whole coconut and use it in a sequence of meals. Coconut cream provides a nice taste to a breakfast or to steamed or stir-fried vegetables.

COFFEE

A cup of coffee as a treat is all right, although it is better to have it black. Coffee has a direct effect on the adrenals to produce adrenaline. Theobromine and caffeine toxins are potentiated through the yeasts used in fermenting coffee. Roasting can also produce carcinogens in coffee.

CORN

Corn (maize) is very protein-rich when eaten fresh. Therefore one should not have corn on the cob with a carbohydrate meal under the 'Hay' system of eating. (This is not the case with tinned corn.)

Corn is a non-glutenous carbohydrate. Cornflakes usually have at least 6 per cent sugar, although there is now a very crispy cornflake without any sugar. It is useful to have Piima yoghourt with the cornflakes or golden linusit (linseeds).

EGGS

It is unfortunate that many people have got used to having a boiled egg with toast as a regular meal; boiled eggs are very hard to digest, the whites of the eggs being particularly hard to break down. Boiled eggs should be heated for five minutes before they are cracked; this destroys an enzyme under the shell so that biotin in the eggs can function normally and reduce any cholesterol risk. Otherwise eat the yolks only.

It is normally better to separate the whites from the yolks as the white part carries most of the mycotoxins from the grains eaten by the birds. (Note that so-called free range eggs are from hens fed at least partly on grains.) And if you separate the whites from the yolks and then beat the whites, they will have a much higher level of oxygen; in other words you will have changed the nature of the protein and made it more assimilable.

If you have irritable bowel syndrome do not have whites of eggs; they take a very long time to degrade in the stomach as they contain a lot of plant as well as animal proteins and a high level of fungus proteins. Yolks are fairly free of contaminants except salmonella or pasteurella.

It is normally acceptable to use whites of eggs in a soufflé, or with cauliflower cheese with beaten white of egg, or you can make a sauce with the yolk, butter and cheese and, when heated, introduce the white of egg and put it under the grill for a short time to brown on top. In this case you would not have destroyed the enzymes which would break down the proteins properly and you would introduce a lot of oxygen when whisking in the egg. You can make a moussaka in the same way – make a fluffy sauce, just putting it under the grill to cook gently on top, when it will be much lighter and easier to digest. Having said that, there is the problem of salmonella to consider so eggs should be purchased from guaranteed salmonella-free laying stock.

FISH

Try to eat only deep-sea fish like whitebait, herrings, anchovies – not mackerel, which are inshore feeders. Try to keep to similar types of food in succession, otherwise the food is going to sit in the stomach for hours: fish and meat require very different enzymes to break them down; on the other hand fish and cheese have similar breakdowns.

Always marinate fish to make it more digestible.

FRUITS

- Mangoes and pawpaws are very enzyme-rich, but the problem is that many are now irradiated so that the sugars are left but the enzymes have been killed. Venezuela, South Africa and Israel all irradiate their fruits.
- Stewing fruit destroys any fungus.
- Grapes, apples and plums all have a very high level of yeast in combination with salicylates.
- Generally, fruit is not recommended for cancer patients because of

the sugar intake. However, for a treat, they can be eaten. It is worth trying to go for a month or so without any fruit and see what difference this makes. (There may be an initial reaction when the toxins are being excreted.)

- Pink grapefruit and any tropical fruits such as avocados, mangoes, pawpaws, lychees, bananas, pineapples and oranges are good. Enzymes such as papain or bromelain found in many tropical fruits can help digest meat, cheese, eggs, etc.
- Fruits break down very quickly in the stomach. If they are eaten close to other foods they will ferment, forming an ideal diet for candida. So be sure to eat fruits at least three hours away from any proteins. Eaten on their own, most fruits pass through the stomach in about half an hour (bananas may take a bit longer).

GARLIC

Garlic and onions are notorious for causing wind. They do this, however, only when they are cooked. Garlic is a bactericide, so it will help move the wind that is there – it does not create it. Garlic can be swallowed with a drink of water; just chop it and swallow it before a meal so that the smell will be lessened, although it still gets into the pores of the skin.

Garlic contains germanium which is one of the most powerful anti-carcinogens, as well as being an antifungal agent.

KELP

Kelp is full of minerals, the B vitamins (particularly B_{12}), and vitamins C, E and K. It also has iodine in a state ready for the thyroid to assimilate.

- It creates surroundings in the intestines that are helpful for beneficial bacteria.
- It reduces pain and swelling of joints, as in arthritis.
- If the heart has been damaged by rheumatic fever earlier in life, kelp will help its action.
- It is useful for people with vague symptoms without any apparent cause as it may provide a missing mineral.

MAYONNAISE

If you use egg yolk to make a mayonnaise, using such ingredients as olive oil, lemon juice, parsley, garlic, then any bacteria in the yolk of the egg will be neutralised. If however you make a mayonnaise with vinegar you will encourage the growth of the pathogens (particularly candida).

If your mayonnaise has been heat sterilised (as in purchased mayonnaises) then the fungi and bacteria which are in the eggs will have been sterilised; however the proteins will also have been denatured, and the body cannot metabolise them properly. It is therefore preferable to make fresh mayonnaise with the yolk (keeping the whites, perhaps with a little bicarb, for use in a soufflé). Should you be concerned about salmonella, cook the eggs and use mashed yolks.

MEAT

Beef has many fungal and other metabolites throughout the meat which do not break down under the heat of cooking. When cooked completely there are no enzymes left, so always marinate meat and only partly cook it. This changes the microflora, and a lot of beneficial bacteria and enzymes that are going to engulf the unwanted bacteria will ensure digestion. When marinating it is best to prick the meat (or fish, for that matter) before marinating so that the lemon juice, etc., gets right into the flesh.

It is preferable, if possible, to have wild game – venison, partridge, pheasant, guinea fowl – which have not been fed on artificial foods.

Avoid ground-up meat if you want to make a sausage or a burger. Grind up the meat yourself, as minced meat from the butcher is very likely to have contamination. This is no indictment of butchers, but the very act of mincing up meat will start the oxidising process.

Avoid pork unless you know how it has been fed.

Avoid pickled meats; marinate them (but not in vinegar) using lemon juice, yoghourt, spices, vitamin C. And avoid processed meats, which will have nitrates, etc., except Parma ham which is cured and which, on analysis, does not seem to have any suspect toxins at all, or excessive salt (some is made from mountain animals never fed on grains).

If you eat lamb, go for New Zealand lamb which will have been free roaming and uncontaminated by Chernobyl fallout. When lamb is not as tender as it should be, mince it with garlic, herbs, yolk of an egg, make it into a little pâté and just lightly grill it without completely killing the enzymes. Once marinated the lamb is far more tender. Lambs' livers should be cut into small pieces and quickly sautéed with a little olive oil to seal them off; they should not be cooked or else they will lose all their vitamins (particularly vitamins B and a high level of K which is very useful in cancer) and it is difficult for the gut to break it down.

Marinate any meats or fish. This predigests and softens the protein and reduces the time needed in actual cooking. This can be done the day ahead and then it only needs a few minutes to heat it, either under the grill or in the oven or wok.

It is always better to go for meat of animals that are not infected with hormones, made-up feeds, with fungi, grains, etc.

MELON

Cantaloupe melons have less sugar and more enzymes than other kinds.

MILK

Cows' milk should not be taken by anyone with a degenerative disease. Cows are usually fed with fungus- or bacteria-infected grain from storage, from big bales and silage. Unfortunately some goatkeepers and shepherds are beginning to give their goats and sheep similar fodder to produce a larger quantity of milk, so some goats' and sheep's milk too is becoming adulterated. Milk is however an important calcium source.

MILLET

This is a non-glutenous grain. Millet is tasty when slightly sprouted and cooked properly; it is also very pleasant in salads. Alternatively, wash it and cook it like rice after soaking it; it separates nicely if cooked very slowly. It can then be mixed with onions, tomato, parsley, garlic, chives, chopped spring onions, etc., or it can be turned into a loaf.

MUESLI

Muesli can be made up of millet and rice flakes, soaked sesame and sunflower seeds, maize flakes (or cornflakes without sugar or malt). There is no real need to have dried fruits in a muesli. Linseed, oat bran and germ can be added.

NUTS

Nuts are heat-sterilised to kill the toxins on their surface. The least contaminated are almonds and hazelnuts, and cashew nuts when they are whole. Broken nuts oxidate easily; walnuts should therefore be bought whole, as the whole nut is generally better – one can see any that are contaminated and throw them out. Walnuts are liable to be contaminated, and are one of the worst for fungus. Similarly buy Brazil nuts whole.

Wash any nuts in hot water and then soak them; this does not make them go soft and flabby, but delicious and much more digestible.

Cooked vegetable and nut mixtures are not very good unless the nuts in them have been soaked. Vegetarians get most of their proteins from nuts and grains, etc., which have not normally been soaked and 'predigested', but are now heat-treated. The only way to get life back into such foods that have been treated – perhaps irradiated – is by washing and soaking them, thus recreating the life forces in them.

In making nut roasts, keep them at a low temperature for a long time, then give them a quick browning to get a crust.

OILS

Sunflower oil, even the unrefined oil, oxidises very fast and does not emulsify well with the saliva. The oils that do not oxidise are olive oil, sesame oil and grapeseed oil.

ORANGE JUICE

Orange juice in cartons often has a certain amount of tartrazine in it. It is not necessary for the producers to declare it on the label as it is used as a production aid (and probably used as a solvent and not a colourant). So anyone with a hyperactive child should not allow them packeted orange juices. (Tartrazine appears to lower zinc levels in hyperactive children.) Tartrazine is also found in golden fish fingers, jellies, ice cream and confectionery.

PARSLEY

Parsley contains iron, vitamins B, C and E, potassium, copper and magnesium, and its digestion time is only 1½ hours.

Parsley tea is good for infections, irritations, congestions and inflammation of the kidneys, bladder, for pyelitis, prostate and any urinary tract problems. Scald a bunch of parsley and cover; when cold, drink over 24 hours. Do this for three weeks. It often works wonders.

PEANUTS

Peanuts consist of starch and proteins, are very acid-forming and indigestible. They are also very prone to mould, whose mycotic secretions (mycotoxins) are carcinogenic. They contain, however, many essential amino acids.

POTATOES

Potatoes without their skins are ordinary carbohydrates: potatoes in their jackets are complex carbohydrates and have a lot of cellulose interlinked with the sugars and starches. Potatoes are rich in potassium and sulphur.

Eating potatoes all the time tends to give one a lot of wind. In the skins particularly there is often a wide range of carcinogens. Potatoes are a member of the deadly nightshade family, and those which have sprouted or are green can be poisonous.

Commercially grown potatoes have antifungicides, pesticides and a high level of nitrates so they are now one of the most contaminated foods; they have also had their sprouts inhibited to give them a longer shelf life. An occasional baked potato will do little harm, and organically grown potatoes are comparatively safe.

Solanine and chaconine, which are glycoalkaloids found in potatoes, are strong enzyme inhibitors and possible teratogens. When plants are bruised, diseased or exposed to sunlight these glycoalkaloids reach levels that can be poisonous to humans. A damaged plant will increase its toxicity as a defence against insects and fungi (a variety bred for its resistance to insects has had to be withdrawn from use because of its toxicity to humans too).

RICE

When rice began to be hybridised the gluten level was increased, so new strains of rice contain much more gluten and starch than the old varieties. The human body, which has evolved over millions of years, has difficulty dealing with these new strains and digests them poorly, allowing *Candida albicans* to proliferate in the gut in response to starches and sugars.

Wash whole rice in clean water. Have rice rather than potatoes. It is better to have non-glutenous grains than glutenous ones, especially for breakfast.

SOUPS

Note that gluten is in all tinned soups as glutamate or modified starch.

SOYA

Soya itself is often contaminated by fungal toxins, so any soya product means an intake of high protein with a level of fungi and plant hormones. A normal healthy gastrointestinal system can cope, but in illness the system is not functioning properly so any aid in the way of curative nutrition must help our metabolic processes to absorb nutrients properly, and any foods that feed candida and other microorganisms should be avoided. Predigested soya in the form of miso or gluten-free soya sauce is all right.

SPROUTED SEEDS

Seeds in general are very full of protein, e.g. sesame seeds contain 20 per cent, sunflower seeds 25 per cent and pumpkin seeds 30 per cent. However, the particular value of sprouted seeds is the increase in the level of vitamins, particularly vitamin C, which reaches a peak about eight days after sprouting. They also have vitamins B2, B6, A, E and K and folic acid. Sprouting changes their carbohydrates into sugars, saturated fats become mainly polyunsaturated, proteins are broken down into their component amino acids; the enzyme action thus makes sprouts easier to digest than dry seeds and beans. They are also a good source of minerals, calcium, iron and chelated magnesium. They can be stored in a fridge for up to seven days, and light cooking can make certain sprouts more digestible still.

Sprouted seeds are therefore one of the richest forms of food. The seedling contains all the future potential of the plant in a concentrated form. The seed's protein is broken down into its component amino acids in a highly digestible form. Enzymes are produced which help in the digestive process. It is as the sprout grows that there is a spectacular rise in its vitamin content and there are also considerable quantities of minerals in the seed itself. Seeds like alfalfa (lucerne) are also highly alkaline at their peak time, and are therefore useful in acidic ailments such as rheumatism and arthritis.

When sprouting seeds, make sure they have been organically grown specifically for food, without any pesticides or fungicides which are normally sprayed on to prevent them from sprouting while stored ready to be planted out the next season.

Seeds can be sprouted in jam jars covered with gauze, but seeds in jars can easily become mouldy and for that reason we would strongly recommend that newcomers to the art of sprouting use the inexpensive commercial sprouters which consists of plastic perforated trays with a lid and water collecting tray. Extra trays can be added so that at any one time there may be four, five, six or more different types of seeds in various stages of sprouting so that it is possible to keep up a regular supply. The work involved in keeping up a supply of sprouts is minimal. They just need to be soaked twice a day, and if sprouting trays are being used this merely means putting them under the running tap until thoroughly soaked. Sprouted seeds can then be available during the whole year and are particularly enjoyable during the winter when there may not be any salad crops in the garden.

Mung beans are probably the easiest seeds to sprout. They can be eaten when they are just showing a minute sprout, or they can be left to grow into sprouts 1 to 1½" long. To grow long sprouts it is best to keep them in a warm area in the dark. Other easy seeds to sprout include aduki beans, alfalfa, lentils, wheat to produce wheatgrass, chickpeas, fenugreek with its curry flavour.

Sprouted seeds can then be eaten in many ways – as fillings for sandwiches, as salads by themselves or with avocados, cucumbers, tomatoes, etc., or they can be lightly steamed or sautéed, or can be combined with other ingredients to make cakes, bread or biscuits.

For further information and recipes using sprouts see *The Complete Sprouting Book* by Per and Gita Sellmann (Turnstone Press) or *Add a Few Sprouts* by Martha H. Oliver (Keats Publishing, USA).

SUNFLOWER SEEDS

These seeds contain 12 minerals, 17 vitamins, 10 amino acids (including all the essential ones), enzymes and pectin. They are full of unsaturated fatty acids, particularly linoleic acid, which is the fatty acid used in preventing deposits of hard cholesterol in arteries, kidneys and the gallbladder.

They are good for skin, bronchial asthma, rheumatoid arthritis and ulcers and, having a lot of vitamins A and B, are good for eye problems. They have plenty of vitamin E and therefore help to prevent blood clots. And the pectin helps to bind and remove radioactive strontium and lead by combining with toxic wastes and forming compounds which can be eliminated.

TEAS

- Pao d'arco tea is particularly good for the liver. It is very bitter, and the hotter it is the worse it tastes. Use it cold out of the fridge three or four times a day.

- Dandelion tea is very bitter; chickweed and sorrel teas are bitter or sour, but very beneficial.
- All normal teas, other than some China tea (which is just dried), go through a fermentation process.
- Earl Grey tea has bergamot in it which is very rich in psoralens which are carcinogenic. (Bergamot is also in one of the leading suntan lotions in France.)
- Kimmun (now with mango) tea and jasmine tea are good.

TOMATOES

- If eaten raw, tomatoes give a very alkaline reaction, but if cooked they are very acidic.
- They are low in calories.
- Minerals include sulphur, salicylates, bromine and cobalt.
- They contain vitamins A, B and C, and all the essential amino acids when eaten straight from the plant.

It is worth noting that if an arthritic person gets a painful reaction after eating tomatoes, it is not because tomatoes are acid but because they are 'stirring up' the stiff joints through the action of the salicylates in them.

WATERCRESS

Watercress is good for protecting against colds, flu and chronic congestive ailments.
- It has vitamins A, B1, B2, niacin and C.
- It also has calcium, iron, chlorine, magnesium, phosphorus and sodium.
- It is good against streptococcal infections.
- Its reaction is highly alkaline; it is therefore useful to counteract an over-acid stomach.

WHEAT

The recommended way to eat wheat is by sprouting it to transform the protein within it into a complete protein, instead of a 'makeshift' protein, the product of several strains. If you sprout it you can make bread and biscuits or Ryvita-type crackers by putting it into a food processor and mincing it well. In the Dead Sea scrolls there is a clear recipe for making bread, which is worth taking to heart. 'Let the angels of air and water bring the life forces back into the dormant grain. Wash it very well, and leave it soaking in the sun until it shoots. Then crush it and let it ferment naturally.' Flavour with salt, herbs, loganberries, etc. and cook at a very low temperature.

YOGHOURT

All commercial yoghourts are made from boiled milk and then that totally inert product is inoculated with live yoghourt. Piima yoghourt made with goats' or ewes' milk seems to be the most beneficial form of yoghourt available (see page 242).

23
NUTRITION AND DISEASE

It is necessary to appreciate that there is no system of feeding that will suit everyone – each person must find out their own kind of diet. One should not look on dieting and eating the right kinds of foods, in the right combinations, as being irksome: it is a challenge and its pursuit can be fun, as well as hard work.

It is unfortunate that often one finds that one's favourite foods are on the list of forbidden foods. This is particularly the case where allergies are concerned, as often one becomes allergic to a food commonly eaten. However, there are always interesting alternatives. It is amazing how one's tastes change or can be made to change. For instance after complete abstinence from sugar in any form for three months or more there will be an instinctive revulsion to anything sweet. Readers who are addicted to chocolate every day may be sceptical, but it is true. It only needs a comparatively short time of struggle, supported by a powerful motive for change, to overcome any form of food addiction.

This is not a recipe book, but there are certain principles of eating that should be understood and, if possible, followed by anyone with a degenerative disease of any kind. It has been said that 'most of the chronic diseases, including cancer, which are prevalent in western countries today, are related to congestion of the metabolic system due to faults in the digestion, absorption and assimilation of food', and, we would add, particularly in the elimination of food residues.

The main metabolic causes of degenerative diseases are:

- Disturbance of the acid/alkaline balance, the pH of the body fluids.
- A diet over-rich in protein and animal and vegetable fats, refined carbohydrates and chemical additives. (It is important to look at vegetable fat as a CAUSATIVE agent in cancer and the motor disorders when it is processed, rancid or laced with antioxidants.)
- The effect of the build-up of a glutenous lining to the small intestines due to the activity of microorganisms, thereby preventing the passage of nutrients through the gut wall into the bloodstream. In this case, however good the diet is, the body is not getting the

benefit of it and this problem should be looked at before assuming that changes in the diet will be of much help.
- Inefficient elimination of waste products.

It is important not to think of changing diet as dieting; the whole concept of dieting is one of restriction, with penalties for breaking the diet. This only adds unnecessary stress to one's already highly stressed life. It is much better to take a positive attitude and find out what suits best, within certain guidelines. Whatever you then choose will make you feel so much better and have an uplifting effect on the quality of your life.

One immediate step to take is to write down all the foods taken over a period of, say, a week, together with a record of any changes in your symptoms to see if there is a pattern of symptoms related to the foods eaten, i.e. whether the symptoms change with the change in foods. Is this a chore, or is it the first step in taking responsibility for your own health?

There is a need to know and understand the implications of what you are eating and why. One man's meat is another man's poison. This is particularly true when people have any form of degenerative disease. People also choose their food to eat on the basis of many different reasons, so these must also be taken into account when choosing a range of foods individually suited to you. For instance there may be moral reasons for not eating eggs produced by battery hens; or there may be a fear of getting too much cholesterol from eating eggs; or eggs may be too expensive an item to include in the family budget.

Besides tailoring one's eating to those foods from which one can benefit, each disease has its own special requirements or taboos. Someone with jaundice cannot tolerate any fats, yet a certain amount of fat is acceptable or even necessary in other ailments. Here again the type of fat is important, so a working knowledge of the benefits or problems associated with certain foods is necessary. Many people have no idea that what they are eating is killing them slowly. And most people overcook their food and turn a nutritious food into a vehicle for carcinogens.

Lastly one needs to know if the food one is eating is being digested properly and its nutrients getting to the places where they are required. Food combining under the system developed by Dr William Howard Hay, known as the Hay diet, is strongly recommended (details are in the next chapter). This system helps to keep food moving so that it does not stagnate and ferment in the stomach.

The principal idea is to allow the body to be programmed to break down whatever comes into it, rather than having to cope with whatever hits the tissues first, as for instance when something like cake is eaten. Here the starches and sugars will set the metabolic clock going, but within the food 'ball' are the undigested proteins and fats (which should have been digested in the acid stomach) which will be carried into the small intestines. Fermentation will then result, with a lot of acidity, even ulceration and tissue breakdown, in the duodenum. All the time the duodenum is trying to break down the undigested foods that should have been broken down in the stomach, but which have been carried into the intestine. People who have followed the Hay diet, as elaborated in the book *Fit for Life* (see page 169), have recorded an increase in energy, loss of excess weight, gradually and permanently, and less gastrointestinal problems. (Some people, of course, can eat anything and have no trouble whatever. They must be able to produce the necessary enzymes all the time.)

In considering an eating plan for sick people, one major change to normal eating habits is cutting down on any products that have toxins in them.

Certain principles are useful to keep in mind:

- Always start a meal with something raw, never anything hot. Hot foods are responsible for the production of excessive mucus. The body recognises something cooked and hot as being something that has started the putrefactive process (and this includes milk that has been pasteurised, which is a process that kills all the lactic enzymes necessary for the body to metabolise it).

- Marinate proteins; this predigests and softens the protein, and helps digestion if the stomach is not producing sufficient acid and if the small intestines do not have enough enzymes to break down any large particles of protein. Use lemon juice, vitamin C, perhaps light yoghourt for marinating chicken or lamb. Once marinated, these meats are far more tender. Marination also neutralises harmful fungal and bacterial toxins.

- Try and find food that has not been contaminated by sprays, artificial fertilisers, hybridisation, and meat that has not been subjected to hormone injections nor been fed with glutenous or infected foods. Venison and animals reared extensively on grass are the best but, unfortunately, in very short supply. However, if naturally reared animals are eaten, this will leave the body some energy for its normal activities and not tie up all its activity with digesting unnatural foods. (Sometimes the body needs so much energy to digest its food that it has not enough left for its tranquillity and peace or to allow it to sleep properly.)

One cannot go wrong in trying to use foods that are easily digested. With any kind of degenerative disease, one has to give one's body the chance to use the nutrients from the food. If you give it food that is hard to break down, you are not helping but hindering your own metabolic processes. If you are very thin, give your body something easy to digest, i.e. proteins that have been predigested or a porridge with very fine grains rather than coarse ones. Pain and discomfort can be significantly lessened when you are soothing the mucosa with gentle food that is easily absorbed.

Always have handy a spray container with vitamin C. This is a powerful antioxidant and counters the oxidising effect of cutting, grating, chopping, etc. Oxidation releases free radicals, which are 'silent killers' of cellular systems. For example, they can be responsible for perforation of the cell wall, resulting in the process known as cell blebbing (leaking of cell contents, which begin to ooze out). During cell blebbing the gene material inside the nucleus of the cell begins to behave in a peculiar manner and its chemical characteristics change dramatically, with the result that normal genes may become cancerous. Clusters of cells then start to grow and pack themselves together, or the cell may atrophy. There may, on the other hand, be a breakdown process (fibrosis) or a hardening process like arthrosis, or ataxia – the illness that develops will depend on the kind of toxins involved.

However, if the lifestyle that resulted in the production of the faulty cells can be reversed, then the genes can be guided to behave normally. It underlines the necessity for good nutrition, purification, cleansing, good air, lessening of stress, etc. It also suggests it is not a good idea, nor may it in the end be found necessary, to poison or cut out or irradiate living tissues.

It used to be thought that, in disease, something was happening to make cells 'go berserk'. Now it is known that a malignant process develops if there is continuous cell damage, of whatever nature, caused by toxins through radiation, drug treatment, or whatever. It is therefore necessary to oxygenate the cells so that cell repair can take place while a person is having surgery, radiotherapy or chemotherapy and to give antioxidants to stop the degenerative process and stop the evolution of an illness. People have to involve themselves in the procedure of change – and remember that healing and a return to normality can take a long time. The cancer cell is not an enemy within, but has been damaged from influences outside itself. The cells which degenerate can regenerate, but this is possible only as long as there is sufficient available oxygen, hydrogen, nutrients etc., which are essential for the cell.

24
THE HAY SYSTEM OF EATING

'Don't mix foods that fight' is the battle cry of devotees of the Hay system of eating. This is not a diet in the conventional sense – there are basically no restrictions on what one can eat (although there are suggestions as to which are the healthier foods to eat), only in the manner in which the foods are combined. It is not the amount of food eaten that is important, but the amount that is properly digested and metabolised by the body. We are not only what we eat, but what we can metabolise properly in order to get the required nutrients. Dr Hay originally wrote about this system in *A New Health Era*, and it has been brought up to date in *Food Combining for Health* by Doris Grant and Jean Joice (Thorsons). The Hay system provides an economical method of eating as all the nutrients from the food digested are released more efficiently into the blood. The body is more easily satisfied so unnecessary extra food, which would normally be stored as fat, is not required. Also, through efficient digestion, less toxins needing to be excreted are formed.

There is one underlying cause of most diseases, i.e. the wrong chemical condition in the body as a result of an accumulation of acid end-products of digestion and metabolism in amounts greater than the body can eliminate. This gives rise to toxaemia, auto-intoxication or self-poisoning.

All one has to remember with the Hay diet is the principle of not mixing concentrated starches with concentrated proteins, i.e. concentrated proteins should not be eaten with concentrated carbohydrates. And that, basically, is almost all there is to it. The reasons for this statement are as follows.

Proteins require an acid medium for digestion and this is supplied by the hydrochloric acid (HCl) and the enzyme pepsin in the stomach. The stomach normally produces as much HCl as is required to digest the amount of protein taken in, but if there are alkaline starches mixed with it, the acidity of the stomach is partially neutralised and is then insufficient to digest the proteins fully. There is not all that much acidity initially in the stomach to interfere with the digestion of alkaline foods or to neutralise the alkalinity of the ptyalin (the salivary enzyme which begins the digestion of carbohydrate) which arrives in the stomach with starchy foods. The acid in the stomach then increases after 30 to 45 minutes during the digestion of food.

Dried legumes (peas, beans, lentils) are the only starchy foods which also contain too high a percentage of protein for their digestion.

Carbohydrates (starches and sugars) require an alkaline medium and therefore need to get passed, as quickly as possible, through the acid stomach into the alkaline medium of the small intestines where the final digestion takes place. Digestion of starches and sugars (carbohydrates) actually starts in the mouth through the action of an alkaline enzyme, ptyalin, which continues to work on the starches as they pass through the stomach. Ptyalin splits carbohydrates into dextroses (or sugars) and this takes half to three-quarters of an hour. If, however, carbohydrates are mixed with the animal proteins then the stomach acid is partially neutralised, which means that the proteins are not fully digested, amino acids are not produced and large toxic molecules of protein are left undigested. These undigested proteins then provide food for fungi and other scavenger bacteria, and some also get passed through the gut wall into the bloodstream undegraded. Where there is a mixture of the two types of food there cannot be complete digestion of either kind of food. In addition, the mixture stays longer in the stomach and the alkalising effect of the ptyalin is reduced or completely neutralised, and the whole mass starts to ferment. Extra histamine (a toxic protein molecule) is produced. Wind, inflammation and constipation or diarrhoea often result.

SOME DEFINITIONS

- Concentrated foods are defined by Diamond as 'any food that is not a fruit and is not a vegetable'. He goes on to say that 'The human body is not designed to digest more than one concentrated food in the stomach at the same time.'

- Carbohydrates (CHO) are made up of carbon, oxygen and hydrogen. Refined carbohydrate constitutes empty calories, e.g. white sugar and flour, semolina, potatoes without skins. These substances do not contain the nutrients to service their utilisation; they are dangerous, robbing the body of nutrients. Unrefined carbohydrates are whole grains, brown rice, peas, beans, lentils, nuts, dried fruits, fruits and vegetables. The less refined the carbohydrate is, the more slowly it is used by the body. This means that the blood sugar levels do not rise appreciably so there is no need for the pancreas to produce extra insulin and there is no danger of hyperinsulinism.

- Fibres are either 'hard' as in bran and grains, or 'soft' as in fruit. A diet of mixed fibres is best. The main advantages of eating sufficient mixed fibres are that you feel more satisfied with a smaller amount eaten, and, more importantly, the fibre helps to clear out the colon and encourages the bowels to move regularly. In particular it helps to move along animal protein so that it does not ferment while lingering in the colon, thus reducing the chances of getting diverticulitis or cancers. It also means there is no straining at stool so there are unlikely to be any haemorrhoids (piles) or varicose veins.

- Proteins constitute some of the largest molecules in the body. They are too large to pass through cell walls, so must be broken down into their constituent building blocks of amino acids before they can be used by the body cells. Proteins that we eat are of plant or animal origin, so their component parts have to be 'rearranged' into human protein before they can be used. Proteins, like carbohydrates, are made up of carbon, oxygen and hydrogen, but also have nitrogen and other elements incorporated into their structures. Nitrogen with hydrogen forms amines (NH_2) and when these amines get attached to carbon atoms they produce amino acids.

- Fats also consist of carbon, oxygen and hydrogen. As they do not mix well with water they can be more difficult to digest than carbohydrates and proteins, both of which are easily mixed with the digestive enzymes. Fats are important sources of energy in the body, but if we eat more than we need they can also form stores of energy, i.e. fatty deposits around the body.

- Vitamins – the word vitamin is derived from vital amines, although not all vitamins are amines. Each individual has his or her own pattern of vitamin requirements and these requirements may vary widely.

- Enzymes are present in every living cell, and carry on the functions of the body, including digestion, waste removal and reproduction. Enzymes are proteins, made from amino acids. Many enzymes are denatured by heat over 104 degrees Fahrenheit. Raw vegetables and fresh fruit are therefore essential for the health of the body's cells as they contain many enzymes and other proteins which have not been denatured by cooking. The ideal to aim at is 60 per cent raw food, but even if this is impossible it is useful to eat something raw before a cooked meal, to help produce enzymes for the digestion of the food to come.

ACID/ALKALI BALANCE

There is one refinement in the Hay system of eating that is important. To maintain the body's correct acid/alkali basis there should be approximately four times as much alkali-forming food as acid-forming food, i.e. 80 per cent alkaline-producing food to 20 per cent acid-forming. To do this means a large intake of vegetables and some fruits (which, although perhaps acid-tasting, are all alkali-forming) compared with the quantity of acid-forming animal proteins and starchy foods (which include skinned potatoes), nuts (except almonds) and sugars.

- Acid-forming foods are all animal proteins and concentrated carbohydrates, such as grains, bread, sugars.
- Alkali-forming foods are all vegetables (including potatoes cooked in their skin, the skins being eaten), all salads, all fresh fruit (except plums and cranberries), almonds, milk.

Keeping proteins and carbohydrates separate does, in practice, help to keep this acid/alkaline ratio steady, as less starchy foods are normally required due to those that are eaten being used more efficiently.

ELIMINATION OF FOOD WASTES

A book that goes further into the principles of the Hay diet is *Fit for Life* by Harvey and Marilyn Diamond (Bantam Books). This is a book for slimmers and includes gluten products and a lot of fruit, so is not aimed at, nor is it completely relevant to, the seriously ill. It does, however, emphasise strongly the need for adequate elimination of food wastes from the body. Each 24-hour period is made up of eight hours during which the main meals are taken (from midday to about 8 pm), eight hours in which the body assimilates what has been eaten (8 pm to 4 am), and eight hours (from 4 am to midday) during which the body is eliminating the residues. During this last period the body should not be using up valuable chemical energy in processing new food while it is taking the necessary action to eliminate waste which, if it were to pile up, would be very damaging to health. It is suggested that nothing but fruit (which passes through the stomach in a very short time) should be taken during this 4 am to midday period. There are however restrictions on the taking of fruit on an anti-cancer diet.

Dr Hay originally suggested that, to achieve his aims, one should have:

- One alkaline meal (preferably breakfast), which should be mainly fruit.

- One carbohydrate meal, such as a salad sandwich or a baked potato and salad.
- One protein meal.

(This fits in neatly with the programme suggested in *Fit for Life*.) Furthermore, Dr Hay also suggests:

- Constipation is a main cause of acid formation.
- Eat only when you are hungry.
- Never eat when tired or mentally upset.
- Do not drink with meals.
- Completely avoid refined carbohydrates such as white flour and sugar, as well as any processed foods.
- Sedentary people should increase alkaline and decrease protein and starch meals.

Anyone following the Hay nutrition programme will lose weight until they arrive at what is, for them, an ideal weight at which they will stick. They will also feel immensely more energetic, with a feeling of well-being. Conversely, an underweight person will, after perhaps an initial slight loss of weight, put on weight until they arrive at what should be their perfect weight.

Although the Hay diet theory is simple, many people find it hard, in practice at first, to keep proteins and starches separate, as this goes against the normal accepted routine. The greatest stumbling block is probably not being able to have potatoes with a meat or fish dish, or a meat, cheese or egg sandwich, or toasted cheese.

THE HAY SYSTEM AND DISEASE

Dr Hay was convinced that many ailments, including the common cold, were a result of disturbed body chemistry. People who have successfully carried out the Hay diet claim it has stopped them from getting colds, has cured eczemas (possibly partly as a result of giving up sugars), helped allergies through production of extra anti-histamines. It will also benefit arthritis sufferers and in fact anyone with a chronic or degenerative disease. All bloating normally ceases after a period in which food combining is conscientiously carried out. It should, however, be realised that it could take up to five years of correct eating to achieve a balanced chemistry in the body, although there are many testimonials from people who have noticed some benefit within days.

- Allergies are often caused by production in the body of histamine (responsible also for hayfever, asthma, migraines, eczemas, urticaria). Yoghourt, provided it is live, eaten daily inhibits the production of histamine, and about three months of combining foods should help overcome allergies.

- Arthritis is an example of a disease where it is best to treat the cause – a deranged chemistry of the body, mainly caused by excessive consumption of starches and sugars.
- Cancers – there is increasing evidence that many cancers are caused by improper diets and faulty lifestyles.
- Common cold – 'Every cold is merely an expression of the body's effort to clean house'. Therefore prevention lies in arranging for the body not to have accumulated waste products in it.
- Dental caries can be prevented by food combining, particularly where food is more alkaline than acid.
- Diabetes – it has been realised that diabetics should eat a high proportion of unrefined carbohydrate foods, and Dr Hay has claimed that his diet has actually cured diabetes.
- Eczemas – all skin problems are external evidence of an internal toxic state from fermentation and putrefaction of incompletely digested carbohydrates and proteins.
- Headaches, except for those caused by sunstroke, excessive noise or an accident to or pressure on the vertebrae, are a result of a toxic state of the body.
- Indigestion, which is often accepted as a normal part of life, often disappears on combining foods.
- Obesity – excess weight can be slowly and permanently removed, without the use of crash diets, calorie counting, artificial appetite suppressants or cutting down on the quantity of food eaten. Obesity is also closely allied to arthritis, constipation, indigestion and heart diseases.

FURTHER READING

Food Combining for Health by Doris Grant and Jean Joice (Thorsons); *Fit for Life* by Harvey and Marilyn Diamond (Bantam Books); *The Bristol Diet* by Dr Alec Forbes (Century).

25
RUDOLF BREUSS AND HIS 42-DAY CANCER TREATMENT

Rudolf Breuss, an Austrian doctor born in 1899, developed the out-standingly successful theory that as cancer needs protein to grow, if you cut out protein the cancerous cells starve and the growth stops. Moreover, protein only needs to be cut out for 42 days, which is the period that the body can survive without any protein at all. During a long enough fast, the body will eliminate everything which does not belong to it. Blood cells can be seen slowly to return to normal during this treatment; through Kirlian photography changes in a person's aura can also be seen in studies of patients on the Breuss programme.

Breuss stipulated that no food should be taken during this period, other than organically-grown vegetable juices, together with herbal teas to keep the kidneys, liver and bowels working properly, plus essential minerals in liquid form. The Breuss vegetable mixture is three-fifths beetroot, one-fifth carrots, one-fifth celery, with a little white radish and egg-sized potato. These juices must be mixed with saliva in the mouth. Drink it slowly with a spoon, consuming up to half a litre a day.

For those without adequate gardens to provide the organically grown vegetables, vegetable juices are available in healthfood shops or direct from the UK agents (Vessen Ltd, Mansen House, 320 London Road, Hazel Grove, Stockport, Cheshire SK7 4RS). Always take the juice with vitamin C to counteract the high sugar content, which would otherwise feed the candida species.

Herbal teas should be taken in conjunction with the juices.

- Sage tea, which Breuss says should subsequently be drunk during the rest of one's life. Take one or two tsps in ½ litre of boiling water, boiled for 3 minutes only; leave to draw for 10 minutes. Drink slowly, and do not swallow straight away.

- Kidney tea, which consists of horsetail (15 g), nettles (10 g), bird knot grass (8 g), St John's wort (6 g). Put a pinch in a cup of hot water, leave to draw for 10 minutes, strain and once again add two cups of hot water and boil for 10 minutes, then strain. Use for three weeks only at the start of the treatment, and as a preventative three or four times during the year.
- Cranesbill tea, particularly after radium treatment, although Breuss does not consider that his treatment will be successful once radium treatment has been undertaken. This tea is to cut out poisons from the body. Add a pinch to a cup of hot water, leave to brew for 10 minutes; have one cold cupful daily.
- Marigold tea, to help cell formation.
- Peppermint tea and/or lemon balm tea can be taken during the whole time of the treatment.

Breuss emphasises that cancer patients who smoke and do not give it up during their treatment will not benefit much, and the treatment would be unsuccessful.

Breuss contends that a cancerous growth is an independent growth that is mainly caused through pressure in the tissues. The point that is pressured wants to live and 'collects from its surrounding the missing materials, causing a growth'. Any surgery on this point subsequently can initiate metastastic growth elsewhere.

FURTHER INFORMATION

See *Cancer/Leukaemia and Other Seemingly Incurable Diseases* and *Advice for the Prevention and Treatment of Numerous Diseases Including Cancer and Leukaemia*, both by Rudolf Breuss. Copies available from Healthfood shops (9 Magdala Road, Nottingham, NG3 5DE) or direct from Walter Margreiter (Im Hag 23, A-6714 Nuziders, Austria).

26
DETOXIFICATION

Detoxification must be carried out first before the body can function properly, particularly since it is very likely that it has been storing up waste since childhood, even since babyhood, due to the passing of toxins through the placenta from the pregnant mother. In children the lymph circulation is often full of toxins, which provide an ideal breeding ground for bacteria and give rise to the childhood illnesses and diseases such as otitis, tonsillitis, sinusitis and other infections. Then there are the adolescent problems such as acne, growing pains, rheumatic fever, eczema, etc., which are all indications of the lymph trying to get rid of its toxins, this time through the skin.

It will be necessary to carry out any detoxification programme for a minimum of three months. The first step in such a programme is to alter one's eating habits in order to have small meals every three hours. This means you do not get bloated with food – the right kind of food in the right combination will not bloat you. This also puts you into a regular rhythm of food intake and helps you regain rhythmical control of glands and nerves. The aim should be to eat food that will be processed immediately in the stomach and intestines, and not to eat foods like sugars that, by their nature, are digested very quickly and then go on to feed tumour cells, or to a place where there is inflammation.

Detoxification can take a very long time; Beata Bishop in her book *A Time to Heal* (Severn Publishers) describes how it took her 18 months of very rigid dieting and detoxification before she could be sure she had overcome a malignancy. The problem is that a cancer is a whole-body ailment, affecting the whole organism in one way or another, and we can never be quite sure that our bodies have become capable of stopping degenerative changes. It is therefore a challenge, with exciting possibilities of actually doing something ourselves to overcome our disability and a feeling that we are not in some way apart from others. It brings about a greater body awareness.

The detoxification programme consists of:

- Fasting initially, followed by a diet with a minimum of yeast, sugars and moulds.

- Coffee or vitamin C retention enemas.
- Cleansing the colon.
- Cleansing the skin.

During detoxification, the body will try to eliminate all its toxins (poisons, including cancer cells) and the blood will be carrying these toxins to the liver and kidneys for elimination. The toxins in the bloodstream will pass through the brain, and this may produce headaches.

FASTING

- Drink at least 3 pints of liquid a day, e.g. lemon juice, grapefruit juice, Breuss vegetable juices.
- Take 100 mg niacin a day. This flushes out toxins from the capillaries and may induce a temporary blushing sensation (the niacin flush).
- Take 2 grams of vitamin C a day.
- Take 50 mg of potassium a day.

After throwing off the toxins and burning all available glucose, the body starts breaking down fatty tissue to supply energy, producing more toxic byproducts which have to be countered by further supplies of vitamins and minerals.

USING ENEMAS

A coffee enema is one of the most potent methods for detoxifying the liver as caffeine goes direct to the liver, stimulating the flow of bile and flushing out toxins. Gerson uses coffee enemas very often in his treatment of cancers, but it is also helpful in the treatment of migraines and arthritis. Coffee taken by mouth has a significant adverse effect on the lymph system and should not be drunk often.

When giving oneself an enema one should try and have sufficient time set by so that there is no stress or pressure to get it done quickly. Get comfortable – have the radio nearby or read a book. With a little planning the period set aside can be calming and peaceful.

The coffee should be prepared beforehand. Use three tablespoons of freshly ground coffee (not instant or decaffeinated coffee) to a quart of water – preferably distilled. Boil (essential) the coffee for three minutes and then stand for at least 15 minutes before straining. Half a pint of this is used when it gets down to body heat, the remainder being readily available for heating up for later enemas.

The simplest device for self-administering an enema is the kind which has a one-way valve in the rubber tube, one end of which is in the coffee water, the other end, after being greased with a water soluble jelly, cream, olive oil, etc., is inserted into the rectum while you lie on your right side with the knees pulled up. Squeeze the bulb, using only enough pressure to get the coffee water in, and repeat until the half pint is used. It's as easy as that.

Then hold the enema in for at least 15 minutes. It is useful during this time to massage your abdomen gently to spread the enema, and to change from one side to the other at times. Enemas have been found quite comfortable when taken in the bath. If you are very constipated it is best to have an ordinary warm water cleansing enema first, and a coffee retention enema an hour later.

Instead of coffee, which under modern methods of cultivation contains high levels of toxic chemicals or fungi, one can use 4 grams of vitamin C powder mixed into 2 pints of distilled water, with 15 ml of zinc, both of which are antioxidants.

Have a retention enema three or four times a week, interspersed with an ordinary water cleansing enema; having fairly frequent enemas means that food does not have time to putrefy in the colon. Above all, look on this as relaxing and not unpleasant, as an essential procedure in the elimination of toxins and for cleansing the liver. It can also give quite amazing pain relief. It is a procedure one can do for oneself, where one does not normally have to rely on anyone else. It does, however, need some planning and self-discipline, but this is a small price to pay for helping in the healing process.

LIVER DETOXIFICATION

Obvious signs of liver toxicity are:

- Chronic constipation; dizziness, inability to concentrate; uncontrolled temper; black offensive faeces; offensive body odour.
- Continuous tiredness, especially in the morning.
- Sallow, aging skin; lines on the face.
- Addiction to sweets, coffee, cigarettes, starches; overeating, or no appetite.
- Stuffy nose, mucus in the throat; acid, bitter or salty taste in the mouth; encrustations around the eyes; wax in the ears.
- Coated tongue.

The processing and excretion of waste products – which will include undigested food particles, excretions of bacteria, dead bodies of bacteria, dead cells, etc. through the liver, kidneys, lungs and skin – is a continuous process.

When toxins enter the blood, the kidneys are the main instrument of elimination (including the excretion of highly toxic polysaccharides). But there is first of all a deposition in the connective tissue, as a temporary storage phase. When this depot is full up, toxins pass into the blood and may result in obesity, arteriosclerosis, varicose veins, calculi, dropsy, cysts, rheumatic nodules, etc.; any tissue that sustains particularly severe damage may finally become malignant.

During treatment of cancer, toxins are released into the bloodstream for elimination and extra debris accumulates in the form of dead cancer cells. This may overload the liver and kidneys, resulting in toxaemia, which is a sign that they cannot cope. The necessary detoxification has to be carried out slowly – often showing up as fever, pain and malaise – otherwise further toxicity will appear. Where liver cells are subject to continuous vitamin deficiency they are unable to counter effectively the daily onslaught of environmental toxins, or cope with internal toxins either.

Gerson has said that before cancer can be controlled, the liver must first be detoxified, i.e. the liver stressed first. If this occurs it will be followed by tumour formation, which in turn makes the liver degenerate even further. Tumours are therefore only an outward sign of a whole body disease.

The liver is thus the main organ of detoxification and is responsible for:

- Metabolising essential fats, preventing their accumulation in the bloodstream where they often form deposits on the blood vessel walls (atherosclerosis).
- Synthesising the bulk of necessary blood proteins.
- Breaking down and eliminating most drugs and environmental poisons.
- Secreting bile, which acts as a carrier for all liver wastes and often, as a result of modern eating, gets clogged up, resulting in the formation of gallstones. As the free flow of the gallbladder slows down there is progressive stagnation and congestion of the liver, resulting in poor assimilation of fat-soluble nutrients leading to psoriasis, eczema, dry skin, falling hair, tendonitis, night blindness, accumulation of calcium in the tissues, prostate enlargement, haemorrhoids.

For cleansing the liver you should take the following:

- Lecithin, daily.
- Apple juice or cider, which acts as a solvent in the bile.

- Epsom salts (by mouth or enema), for its magnesium, to relax the muscles of the bile duct.
- Olive oil (or another unrefined oil) to stimulate the gallbladder to contract powerfully, thus expelling solid particles which may have remained there for years.
- Vitamin C or coffee retention enemas (see p. 173 for procedure).
- Caraway seed enemas are also helpful. Infuse two spoonsful in 2 litres of water; use tepid, not hot.

CLEANSING THE COLON

Often such drugs as antibiotics kill the friendly bacteria in the colon (large intestine), e.g. the acidophilus or bifidobacteria, allowing them to be replaced by disease-causing organisms (such as candida) which produce ptomaines, leading to a low-level chronic form of ptomaine poisoning (homoeopathic ars. alb. may be helpful here).

Low-fibre meals make it more difficult for the colon to eliminate wastes; high pressures are required for squeezing remnants of low-fibre meals through the colon, and these may cause blowouts in the colon wall (diverticuli). Therefore you should eat a high-fibre diet.

The colon should be slightly acid. Foods required to keep it in an acid condition include:

- Acidophilus yoghourt, Piima yoghourt, lactic acid fermented foods. (Note that acidophilus can convert milk sugar (lactose) into lactic acid.)
- Lemon juice in a little water after meals will help maintain a proper acid/alkaline balance.

CLEANSING THE SKIN

The skin is another important organ of detoxification and may become overloaded with toxins as healing progresses and as the body attempts to throw off its accumulated wastes. This may result in skin eruptions, odours, colours, blemishes, etc. Note that if the scurf rim in the iris is very dark, it means the skin is relatively blocked as an organ of elimination.

- 'Skin brush' up the front and down the back of body.
- Have a warm shower and rub with a loofah.
- Sit in a bath of water to which you have added a cup of apple cider vinegar to restore the acid covering of the body.
- An epsom salt bath will help to draw toxins out of the skin.

- Once a week rub a mixture of olive oil and castor oil all over the body. Then have a hot soaking bath for 15 minutes, go to bed and sweat out poisons for an hour, then have a cleansing shower.

OTHER MEASURES

- Raw garlic has a high concentration of selenium and germanium, which help to remove metals such as cadmium, mercury, lead and aluminium.
- Apple pectin and alfalfa sprouts help remove radiation toxicity built up from other foods, e.g. strontium 90 in milk.

Pyretotherapy is the induction of high fever which can increase the number of leucocytes (defence cells used in swallowing up toxins and dissolving them). The resulting inflammation is the body's way of attempting to get rid of toxins (unwanted substances, fungi, bacteria or viruses), but this natural response is often stifled (by antiobiotics and steroid treatment) so the toxins the body is trying to get rid of will be stored, which in turn compromises the immune reactions.

Cancer cells are damaged at a temperature of 105°F, while healthy cells are only damaged at 109.5°F. Fevers therefore weaken cancer cells, and can be induced (by drugs, ultra-short-waves, hot baths,etc.) to kill the cancer cells. (Note that this depletes the body of potassium, which has to be replaced.)

HEALING CRISES

Healing crises (or toxic reactions) may follow detoxification as toxins are dumped into the system and the body begins to heal itself. These may appear as loss of appetite, nausea, headaches, fevers, a sick feeling, listlessness, lack of energy, swelling of various lymph glands. A large amount of toxins is released into the bloodstream which goes to the liver, for removal by way of the bile. This bile is jet-sprayed into the intestines and, if not cleared through the system, will be reabsorbed and go back to the liver, thus overloading it.

In general, cleanse the body by relieving any constipation and make all organs of elimination more active. It is also useful to massage the feet daily as there are nerve connections from the feet to all organs of the body, and massaging stimulates these nerves and helps the relevant organs, as well as toning up the neurovascular system so that it pumps the blood round the body more effectively.

SUMMARY OF DETOXIFICATION PROCESS

- Caffeine irritates the liver, which releases bile into the gallbladder more quickly. Toxic materials are released into the blood system. These circulate and cause flu-like feelings, muscular pains, dizziness, weakness, fainting spells, intestinal spasms, cold sores, as well as inflammatory processes, e.g. pain in and around tumour masses, aggravation of symptoms, rashes.
- Note that dark stools and fever are good signs that the body has become very efficient at detoxification.

The detoxifying process can be used to heal the body of any degenerative disease. The body does not heal selectively – when the body's ability to heal itself is restored, it sets about healing itself of whatever is wrong with it.

27
PAIN CONTROL

Pain naturally has physiological causes, but it can also be caused merely by emotional stress. Therefore not only a person's physical state but also his emotional state must be considered when dealing with his pain.

People with serious diseases, particularly cancer, are often terrified by pain, even the slightest pain, thinking that what to a normal healthy person would only be an ache or a crick in the neck may be the start of further disease, a sign perhaps that cancer has recurred or erupted elsewhere in the body (metastasised).

It is often difficult to tell whether a person's pain is a physical one or the result of some psychological cause. Pain overtly reminds everyone else that one is suffering, needs sympathy, etc. This is called an external reward of pain. An internal reward of pain may be its substitution for some emotionally painful conflict which is difficult to face. If an illness has unconsciously benefited a person, perhaps through a reduction in some commitment or responsibility, then any diminution in that benefit may lead to increased pain, in an effort to regain the lost benefit.

Some people are awakened from deep sleep by intense pain. This may be because the unconscious tends to deal with unpleasant issues during sleep, issues that a person may think are too frightening to confront while awake. The resulting unpleasantness in the dreams results in physical pain.

Pain is thus closely linked to tension and fear. Therefore the relaxation/imagery process, if used properly and regularly, will help reduce muscle tension (thus reducing pain) and may lessen the underlying fear, thus reducing tension still further.

Pain is never constant; there are pain-free moments, moments when the pain is minimal, and times when it varies in intensity. Why? Maybe, unconsciously, we have contributed to an increase in, or the initiation of, pain, through the kind and nature of our thoughts. This realisation of how we may have contributed to our own pain is an important first step in reducing it.

MENTAL IMAGERY FOR COPING WITH PAIN

- Visualise the body's power to heal, through relaxation and whatever imagery one may find the easiest; for example, you might mentally mobilise the white blood cells to overcome the disease which is causing the pain.

- 'Communicate' with your pain through your subconscious or inner guide. Make your pain an entity with whom you can have a dialogue, to find out what purpose it serves. This will soon show whether the pain is being used as an excuse for something – for getting out of a commitment, for increasing one's importance, as a cry for sympathy and attention, etc.
- Substitute pleasure for pain. Deliberately engage in some pleasurable activity. This has been found to decrease pain, albeit temporarily, but it shows that it can be done.

SOME AIDS TO PAIN RELIEF

- Non-steroid anti-inflammatory drugs (NSAIDs, e.g. aspirin, ibuprofen, sulindac, indomethacin, benorylate) are routinely given to relieve pain and reduce inflammation, although the British Medical Association (BMA) are now querying whether NSAIDs may be contributing to progressive disease and long-term damage. They should be given only in the last resort. NSAIDs may help rheumatoid, but not osteo-, arthritis. They inhibit prostaglandin production, so white cells proliferate and cause damage. The side effects of NSAIDs therapy are bowel bleeding, duodenal ulcers, diarrhoea, damage to bone joints and tissues, damage to kidneys and the liver.
- If much of the pain is in the form of headaches one can use pure aspirin or Weleda's Bidor 5.
- Aspirin is also useful if blood thinning is needed alongside pain relief, as it combines both these properties.
- Germanium helps 'scavenge' free radicals (toxic highly reactive molecules with an unpaired electron), its electrons interacting with the free radical's electron. It helps keep up glutathione levels in the body. It is a natural pain reliever.
- Selenium reduces pain levels.
- Cod liver oil often helps. It contains eicosopentaenoic acid (EPA), which helps reduce inflammation.
- Green lipped mussel from New Zealand relieves 60–70 per cent of arthritic pain or headaches.
- The herb feverfew also helps some, but not all, arthritic pain or headaches.
- Vitamin C (10 g intravenously) helps kill pain in terminal cancer.
- Paracetamol is used widely in pain relief. However, it contains a

high level of aluminium; therefore many elderly people who take a lot of paracetamol often show signs of senile dementia with Alzheimer's disease because their tissues show a higher than normal level of aluminium, which is toxic to the body and the brain.

- Reflexology is a system of healing based on breaking down the congestion in organs by manipulating areas on the toes, soles, top and sides of each foot (or hand) which have been found to correspond to different organs and parts of the body. This is a very ancient art, practised by the Chinese (and probably the Egyptians in about 3000 BC). Pressure on these areas reduces pain in the organs to which the areas relate. It is suggested that readers contact a qualified reflexologist who can demonstrate to them how they can treat themselves, or how they can get their partner to treat them.

PAIN CONTROL AND NUTRITION

The nutritional implications of pain control are many and varied, but with sensitive nutritional manipulation it is possible to allay up to about 60 per cent of most pain. Indeed, in many people up to 90 per cent of all their symptoms vanish. However this is not simply a result of diet, but of getting ready to receive the right food at the right time, in the right place and in the right combination. It is a new way of living.

In order to make the best use of the foods we consume it is necessary to get the body organised so that the correct biochemical reactions are followed in the correct order: how to breathe properly; provide oxygenation at a certain time; nerves must send the right messages to the right places; the blood must quicken. We then become procreators, creators, part of our own healing process.

It is a major problem to get through to people that nutrition (and not merely feeding) is an answer to their problem, but they are often not prepared to follow a new simple regime, saying 'I know what you say is right, but I am not prepared to change.' Here in the west we eat much too much, and we tend to eat far too many varieties of foods all at once, with the result that our bodies are overloaded, stressed. In such a situation the body becomes functionally inaccurate at handling all the different categories of foods correctly; it no longer recognises when the nerves have to ring the alarm bells and when they should be silent, nor when the organs should open or close, nor when the glands should secrete materials or not. By the time we acquire an illness our bodies have thus already gone through long periods of such physical and psychological stress. Our culture fixes the way we eat; we get into a habit, a routine, which is very hard to break out of. This is why one of the aims of Springhill is to work with the young because their patterns are not so fixed.

Because of the habitual nature of our lives people ignore symptoms (of allergies in particular); they have become too familiar. But these symptoms are precursors to pain, and action should be taken as early as possible to forestall further development of an ailment that may bring great pain. A simple change in the style of living and eating can often accomplish this. It is useful to start off with a basic set of rules, and then a person can branch out and start experimenting for himself. For example, it is quite amazing how much pain is relieved when there is a flushing out of toxins from the body, while lymphoedema (swelling of the lymph glands) is one of the conditions directly manipulated by nutritional changes. Fluid retention, wind, constipation and bloating are all much related to the way different foods are combined in our diet, and whether or not the body can make proper use of the nutrients from the food.

Supposing you have migraine – at what stage should you think about nutrition? How can you make sure that your food is adequately broken down, that the nutrients from it are actually getting to the tissues that need them, that the eliminative processes are working satisfactorily and there is no putrefaction in your body? Or supposing you have bursitis or muscular pain, sciatic pain, pain under the arm because the lymph nodes are congested, pains from tumours, in the lung or chest, perhaps pains in the liver, which may be overloaded with pathogens, making for an inflammatory condition like chronic hepatitis? These are responses to offending triggers in whatever we take through the food chain or from the environment.

For those who are terminally ill, pain control through nutrition can also be applied. For a start, the lighter the body is, the less need there is of pain relievers. Small, light meals should be taken often; light meals that are easily broken down and digested make for far less pain. Wherever there is a tumour or inflammation or toxicity, then neurological pain is created and the energy through the nerves will be blocked, and the pain will be acute. Reduce the load, mobilise metabolic function, speed up the neurological energy, and there will be very little pain.

With sensitive nutritional manipulation there are so many opportunities to inhibit pain and to lure your neural broadcasting system into not sending wrong messages. It is therefore important for people who are ill and people living with them to know and understand the principles of how things interact and how they are mixed so that the body will itself be able to decide what is needed and send it through to the tissues, and to excrete and eliminate what is not required. This enables our own body wisdom to do the job, to do away with the stresses of wondering what should be done – 'What on earth have I got to do?' is a familiar first reaction to the news that we have some disease or other. And one of the most important answers is that it is essential to have a basic knowledge of nutrition, and of our functional organism.

28
EXERCISE

Death rates from cancer among people having occupations involving the least muscular effort have been shown to be higher than in those occupations involving heavy muscular effort. Dr Hans Selye suggests that this may be because stress may be relieved through exercise, through having a physical outlet for releasing the stress. Vigorous exercise tends to stimulate the immune system.

The act of setting aside time for regular exercise not only indicates a willingness to take charge of one's health, thus contributing to the quality of life; it also creates the emotional climate necessary to help overcome stresses and, coincidentally, relieve pain. Whatever the state of a person's health, it should be possible for them to find some form of exercise, however minimal, that they can perform without injury or stress.

Exercise of any kind generally:

- Improves the circulation.
- Reduces high blood pressure.
- Strengthens the heart and lungs and reduces the chance of heart attacks.
- Reduces blood glucose levels.
- Reduces loss of calcium from bones (osteoporosis).
- Relieves stresses, which are a major enemy of a healthy immune system.
- Increases the levels of endorphins which are brain hormones that create a feeling of well-being.

In considering exercise for people who are ill in any way, it is important to emphasise that they should exercise within their limits and never push themselves beyond that point; otherwise they will only add to their stress. The idea is not to aim for a gold medal in the Olympics. Early morning exercises should be designed for mental and physical destressing, relaxing, loosening muscles and rejuvenating the nerve endings. This will, in itself, extend one's limits over a period of time. The exercises should be simple and uncomplicated, requiring little concentration.

Exercises which are aimed at relieving stress help glandular functions and promote the correct secretions. This is most important in the battle against cancer and other illnesses. People who have been constantly and nervously on the go all their lives are likely to have had their adrenal glands pumping out hormones 24 hours a day; they will not be able to feel rested even in the morning because the adrenals are still pumping. They feel as if they have lead weights or pins in the muscles which feel heavy.

The process of healing is only possible when the body has the chance to rest, the chance to mobilise itself through gentle exercise and proper breathing, and to replenish itself with proper food which is metabolised properly. It is not necessary to jump out of bed and go into a gymnasium for a workout; it is quite possible to do breathing and stretching exercises in bed. At the same time it is often useful to have a background of very pleasant music, or a sequence of sounds (there are many excellent relaxation tapes on the market).

Decide what the body wants to do spontaneously. You should be looking for automatic movements which reflect the body's rhythms in order to clear the neurological pathways, to increase circulation and increase the flow of lymphatic fluids. In this system you do not practise any pre-established movements, but try to get back rhythm and automatic movement. These exercises do have a very practical outcome for people in pain; if the flow of nerve sensory messages is allowed to bypass the area where there is any inflammation, then the pain goes. The simplest exercises are the best. They do not have to be complicated.

- It is a good idea to start the day off with a good stretch – even if you are in bed or on a chair. Stretch like a baby; this stimulates all the sensory nerves.
- Roll from side to side as babies do in their cots. Cradle your legs and rock back and forth. Try to become a child; do the kind of movements that babies (and cats) do when stretching and rocking. This all gets the blood flowing, the spine stretched, nerve impulses working, and mobilises much vital energy to release any parts of the body that are 'locked up'. On a cold morning these exercises can even be done under the quilt, so there is no excuse.
- Breathe in at the same time as you stretch. The object of breathing exercises is to get the breathing rhythm back to normal so that every cell gets adequate oxygen again; 20 to 30 continuous breathing exercises are necessary.
- At rest a person only breathes in and out about a pint of air. The

lungs can, however, hold a gallon (although they cannot exhale the last pint). All cells need oxygen and therefore if one increases one's input of oxygen, even marginally, it will benefit the body's cells. Therefore use the whole breathing apparatus, including the muscles of the abdomen, to move the diaphragm, thus increasing the volume of the lungs and causing more air to be inhaled.

- Yawn. This gives a tremendous amount of nerve stimulation and within a few minutes can change the rate of peripheral circulation.
- Try to make some of the exercises comic so that you have a good laugh. Laughter is the best medicine. Laughter is an emotional catharsis – it does to the mind what enemas do to the body. Share the exercises with someone if possible, even over the phone.
- The whole of the spine must be exercised, while breathing in. Use 'cross crawling' movements in order to unblock the nerve sensory functions, i.e. move the left arm with the right leg, right arm with left leg, etc.
- Get a sequence of movements like swimming; the bath is an ideal place to do these.
- Even when driving a car some exercises can be done.
- Supposing there is a tightness across or round the shoulders, as we all experience from time to time under physical or mental stress. Put both arms just behind the ears and stretch the arms upwards (a very natural movement of stretching for static desk-bound people). Groan at the same time. (If anyone has seen farmhands at work in the fields, one will appreciate the stress-releasing properties of loud groans and grunts accompanying every stroke of the hoe; world-class tennis players resort to grunting when they really put an effort into a shot.)
- For another simple exercise lie on the floor and hook your feet under some weighty piece of furniture so that there is a bit of traction. Get in some really deep breathing. Exercises combined with breathing techniques to release emotional tension often make an enormous difference.
- If the shoulders have a lot of stress and tension in them, tell yourself to lower the shoulders, relax them, and release the tension.

There are of course ailments where energetic exercise may be positively harmful, as in ME, and it is in such cases that a sequence of gentle movements, combined with an awareness of one's body, is so valuable. It is useful to learn something about eurythmy and combine this with the techniques of Dr Feldenkrais, who taught a system called awareness through movement.

THE FELDENKRAIS METHOD

Feldenkrais was an Israeli neurophysiologist specialising in pain control who understood that pain happens in steps, sequentially, and that we can develop a capacity to influence pain through the ways in which our body behaves – our posture, gestures and in the ways our skeletal and muscular frame is held. He taught that one should not only listen to the body, but really find the responses in the body that are purely automatic, which we have ignored. These will be different in each individual. It is useful to learn his theories in the case of any degenerative disease causing pain, such as cancer, arthritis, MS, etc., as his exercises are intended to reduce effort in movement and to eliminate all superfluous movements.

The way we hold ourselves will depend on our self-image, so an improvement in our ideas about ourselves can have a positive effect on our capacity to influence pain. Coue's autosuggestion comes in very handy here (see p. 198). Whatever we can do well seems easy to us and builds up the positive self-image: conversely, building up our self-image will improve our performance. Success breeds success.

However, we do not normally develop our skills beyond a certain low-to-average potential; our self-image is, in the great majority of people, satisfied with this level of attainment. 'We tend to stop learning once we have mastered sufficient skills to attain our immediate objective.' This is partly limited by the type of social environment we each live in; people are satisfied (i.e. they are living up to their self-image) with a limited ability or level of attainment, provided it is acceptable in their level of society. For example, a cabinetmaker will have far higher standards to achieve for his own self-esteem than an amateur who merely wishes to build a set of shelves.

Feldenkrais concluded that 'Natural practices have gradually given way to acquired methods' and society forces people to follow the acquired methods, i.e. people adjust to what is socially acceptable at the time. However, it is important to try and live in accordance with one's natural constitution; man must become aware of how he can move freely. Children illustrate this point well; if they are allowed to develop at their own pace in their own way, they are more likely to develop in accordance with their individual abilities, whereas, in children who are judged primarily by their achievements, all spontaneity will disappear at an early age.

Furthermore, what we learn is very much influenced by what we have learnt in the past. An Englishman may find a French accent difficult to achieve, yet it is 'child's play' to a French child. 'Every pattern of action or learning that has become fully assimilated will interfere with the patterns of subsequent actions.' Habit is behind most actions, and it makes new action difficult to acquire.

Generally humans cease to develop their ability to adjust to circumstances at the age of 13 or 14. Activities of the brain, of the emotions and the body that are still difficult then will remain permanently beyond the bounds of the individual. Repeated unsuccessful attempts to do something will usually make a person abandon that activity and set limits on what they think they can do. This negative feeling may then spill over into other activities, i.e. the self-image is undermined. But success breeds success; movements then become easier, resulting in less tension and greater ease and sensitivity.

Feldenkrais postulated that when we are awake there are four states – sensation, feeling, thought and movement. Most of these states are used all our waking life, so correction of any one will affect the whole body. The easiest and main means of improving the self-image is movement – which involves muscular activity. However, the fact that we actually take some action does not mean we know what or how we are doing it. It takes considerable effort to know what we are doing, in detail.

Muscular activity results from a series of impulses from the nervous system; muscles cannot work until activated by these impulses from the nervous system. But they can also be stopped from working; there is a very short delay between thinking and doing, and this delay gives us time to change our mind and not take action.

Thinking, feeling and moving are thus intimately interconnected. We cannot move without first thinking of what muscles we want to move and in which direction, with what force and for what reason, even though the actual muscles to be used are chosen unconsciously. Continued use of certain muscles will increase the percentage of the brain used to produce these particular muscle movements, e.g. a singer will have more of his brain developed to use the muscles of his chest and throat in a particular way.

Feldenkrais maintained that 'Movements reflect the state of the nervous system which organises muscular movements, which cannot function without nervous impulses to direct them.... Our breathing reflects every emotional or physical effort and every disturbance, every change of strong feeling or anticipation of a strong emotion.'

At a practical level, the skeletal structure should counteract the pull of gravity by itself, without help from the muscles, which are then free to move the body as desired. But in most people certain muscles are always unconsciously at work, e.g. the muscles of the jaw, of the eyelids, of the neck. The aim is to get muscular effort transmitted through the bones, leaving the other muscles free to do their proper jobs. Unnecessary effort, i.e. excess tension, causes the spine to be shortened, for example. Voluntary movements are reversible: involuntary ones are not, e.g. the knee jerk reflex. It is important to learn to turn strenuous jerky movements into smooth and easy ones.

For details of suggested exercises (some of which may be beyond the scope of the elderly or people with stiff joints), see *Awareness Through Movement* by Moshe Feldenkrais (published by Penguin Books).

29
MASSAGE OF ACUPUNCTURE MERIDIANS

Traditional Chinese medicine is based on the concept that there is a life force in all of us called *ch'i*, or *ki*, which flows round the body in a harmonious, balanced manner and that any interruption of this flow causes illness. When this life force is flowing properly there is harmony and health; if it is not flowing properly there is illness. Symptoms of illness are, to the Chinese, signals of distress and pointers to the site of interruption in this flow of life force.

This life force flows round the body in defined pathways, called meridians, which are named after major organs. However an imbalance in the meridian does not necessarily mean there is something wrong with the organ concerned; it may mean something is wrong with a person's lifestyle, or with a facet of their personality. These meridians have been measured and mapped by various scientific methods and can be felt by a trained acupuncturist, who treats various specific acupuncture points along the meridians (again, detectable by electronic instrumentation) in order to release any energy blockage in the meridian. Imbalances in the meridians can be detected by feeling the deep as well as the superficial pulses (to gain an ability to do this may take many years) or through muscle testing under the Touch for Health system.

Touch for Health is a preventative form of medicine aimed at overcoming minor imbalances in the body. When the body's energies are balanced, many aches and pains, allergies, and even some acute and chronic conditions are alleviated. It is a system of applied kinesiology and requires a therapist to apply it to a patient. There are, however, aspects of the system which can be quickly learnt, and, in particular, simplified ways of relieving tension in muscles which a person can follow out by himself or herself.

Some muscles are intimately connected with specific organ systems – perhaps they share a lymph system or an acupuncture meridian. Any blockages in these pathways indicate a weakness in the associated organ system, so any help given to the muscle system by restoring a flow of energy in it also gives relief to the organ(s) which share that meridian.

It is impossible in a book of this size to go further into the theory of acupuncture or Touch for Health. However, there are simple procedures that anyone can learn for helping to maintain a free flow of *ch'i* round the meridians, and these also help in pain relief.

Everything in nature is, to the Chinese, a result of the interplay of two elements, yin and yang; for instance, the solid organs in the body are considered to be yin, while the hollow organs are yang. There are also yin and yang polarities within the body. The Chinese concepts of yin and yang are applied to the flow of energy along the direction of the meridians. Yin energy flows from the earth, i.e. from the feet up the front of the body to the torso, followed by other meridians going along the inside of the arms on to the fingers (looking at the body at all times as if the hands were raised, as in the drawings on page 194). On the other hand, yang energy flows from the sun, so the yang meridians run from the fingers down the outside of the arms to the face, and then from the face down the outside and back of the body to the feet.

There are two techniques developed by the Touch for Health Foundation which will help to keep the energy flow balanced:

- Trace the meridians with the flat of the hand an inch or two above the surface of the body. To sceptics who may think this sounds too far-fetched I would say try it and see the results. There is a continuous flow of energy round the body and therefore it is necessary to treat these meridians in the order specified. Start at the beginning of each meridian and follow the direction of flow. Then trace against the flow. Do these tracings a few times for each meridian, always ending with a trace in the correct direction of flow.

- Massage gently along the line of the meridian in the correct direction of the flow and at the same time think deeply over any tender spots that the meridian passes over. This is one way of unblocking the meridian energy which may have become blocked. Definite statements of a feeling of getting better, even more than merely an intention to get better, can be extremely effective (see page 198 on autosuggestion).

Choose the meridian to work on by relating it to any problem you have in a particular organ, or by locating a painful area and working on the nearest meridian to pass over the spot.

You may wish to use these two techniques on all the meridians as a general 'toning' of the system, or you may wish to use them only on the

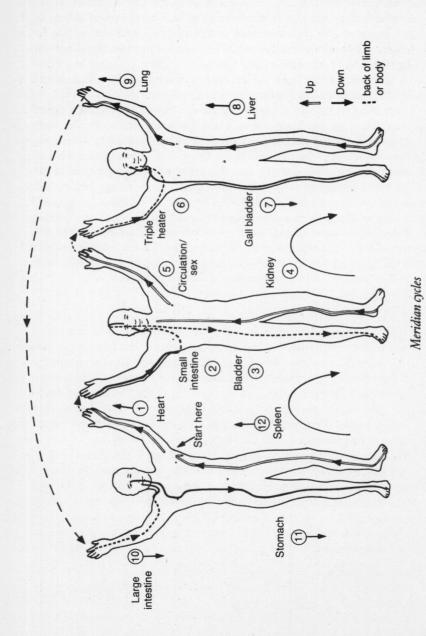

Meridian cycles

meridian intimately concerned with your particular problem. It will probably depend on how much time you wish to spend on getting well.

The meridian pathways look complicated, but once they are learnt there will develop a rhythm in their tracing. They can be traced on you by someone else equally effectively.

There are three main cycles, each covering four meridians, making up the complete flow of energy round the body. The full circle of yin and yang massage from fingertip to face, to feet and back again has to be repeated, with slightly differing pathways, three times in order to cover the whole 12 meridians. To get the full benefit it is suggested you repeat the whole cycle several times once a day – probably after a bath is the best time, when one can concentrate without fear of interruption. These pathways, simplified for quick self-administration, are shown on the accompanying diagrams.

There are also minor meridians – two of which, the central and governing, are mentioned below – with specific functions, but beyond the scope of this book. From the diagrams it will be seen that the meridians in many cases are very close together.

The meridian cycles are in the following order:

- First cycle:
  1 Heart meridian – from chest down the inside of the arm to the little finger.
  2 Small intestine – from the back of the little finger up the outside of the forearm, up the back of the upper arm to the cheek.
  3 Bladder – from above the eye, over the head and down the back and the back of the legs, the outside of the foot to the little toe.
  4 Kidney – from under the foot, the inside of the ankles, up the inside of the leg, straight up the front of the body and up to the collar bone.
- Second cycle:
  1 Circulation/sex – from the chest, down the middle of inside of the arm to the tip of the middle finger.
  2 Triple heater (or triple warmer) – from the outside of the fourth finger, down the outside of the arm, up the neck to the side of the face.
  3 Gallbladder – from behind the ear, down the back of the head, across the front of the shoulder to the armpit, down the side of the body to the fourth toe.
  4 Liver – from the big toe up the centre of the inside of the leg, up the body up to the chest.

- Third cycle:
  1 Lung – from the nipple, up the inside of the arm to the thumb.
  2 Colon (or large intestine) – from the outside of the first finger, down the outside of the arm to the shoulder and up to the upper lip.
  3 Stomach – from the eye down the front of the face to the nipple and straight down the middle of the leg to the second toe.
  4 Spleen – from the big toe up nearly the centre of the leg to the chest, ending below the armpit.

There are two further meridians of importance: the central meridian, going from the centre of the pubic bone, up the front of the body to a point under the lower lip; and the governing meridian, going from a point under the tail bone, up the spine, over the top of the head and down the face to the centre of the upper lip.

It should be remembered that, with the exception of the central and governing meridians, the meridians are on both sides of the body, although, for ease of illustration, meridians on only one side are shown. Both sides should be traced and/or massaged, either simultaneously where possible or one side after the other. When tracing lines at the back of the body it is quite in order to trace one half as far as the arm can reach and then change the arm's position to trace the other half.

The same effect can be reached purely by meditating on the flow of energy round the meridians, again in the specified sequence. Once the pathways are familiar through tracing them with the hand, one has to just think of the flow of energy, using imagination to strengthen the thought and to feel the flow. This of course requires a lot of concentration at first. While concentrating, hold your hands with thumbs folded inside the palms. This meditation has several benefits:

- The deep concentration necessary will dissipate any negative thoughts of pain, worry, depression, anxiety, etc. As Coue says, you cannot think (certainly not deeply) of two things at the same time.
- It is a system of self-healing. Increasing the flow of energy will help to free blockages that may have arisen and which may be the focus for disease.
- By strengthening the flow one is preventing blockages.
- It may be possible, when competent in the meditation, to diagnose any imbalances or blockages which might lead to illness or may be the cause of a present illness, both in oneself and, ultimately, in others. By concentrating on sites in the body where energy has become blocked it is possible to re-establish an unimpeded flow of energy at that point.

By following this system of increasing the subtle flow of energy round the body, anyone with a malignancy or degenerative disease is at least taking some of the responsibility for their own welfare and that, in itself, is a healing process.

Emotional stress release can also be accomplished by oneself in two other ways.

- Just put your fingertips on the frontal eminences of your forehead (called the neuro-vascular points), halfway between the eyebrows and the hairline, and talk yourself through the problem two or three times. This is an excellent method for releasing fears, frustrations and many mental and emotional strains.
- Auricular exercise – as the ears seem to function as 'antennae', drawing energy into the body, firmly take hold of, and unfold as you do so, the turned over part of the ear. Pull firmly away from the opening of the ear, pulling away from the orifice. Do this a few times.

Any method of reducing the effects of stress is worth trying by anyone with a major disease.

USEFUL ADDRESSES

Touch for Health Foundation in the UK, contact Brian H. Butler, 39 Browns Road, Surbiton, Surrey KT5 8ST, tel. 081-399 3215.

30
AUTOSUGGESTION AND THE METHODS OF EMILE COUE

The subconscious consists of the memory of things that have made an impression. It is the inspiration for conscious thought, and all conscious thought is based on action by the subconscious. It is the supervisor of physical processes and accepts all strong impressions it is given. This implies that by conscious thought we can affect the subconscious, which will, in turn, later affect our conscious thought. For instance, any conscious thoughts of fear of falling produces involuntary movements which will make you fall; thoughts of stage fright produce speechlessness and forgetfulness; of embarrassment produce blushing; while thoughts of erotic actions produce physical sexual reactions.

Autosuggestion, as elaborated by Emile Coue, is therefore:

- Acceptance of an idea by the subconscious.
- The transformation of this idea into a physical reality.

To ensure acceptance of an idea by the subconscious:

- Every idea is charged with some emotion. The greater the emotion, the more likely will it be impressed on the subconscious.
- If there is a conscious effort of will to get the subconscious to accept an idea, this will only bring up counter-thoughts.

Where the will and the imagination are in conflict the imagination always wins.

If the mind dwells on the idea of an accomplished fact, the subconscious will produce that state, e.g. if a tennis player has a great will to win, he will play worse and worse under the dominant thought in his imagination of failing. Golfers are afraid they will slice their drive; the will is to send the ball straight, but the imagination is afraid of slicing it, so the muscles obey the imagination.

AUTOSUGGESTION AND HEALTH

If we continually think of happiness we become happy; if we think of becoming healthy we become healthy, i.e. our thoughts become an actual condition of our lives. We can therefore make:

- Particular suggestions, which should give the promise of an immediate start in the desired direction; of rapid progress, ending in complete and permanent cure.
- General suggestions, e.g. every night and morning say, at least 20 times, 'Day by day, in every way, I'm getting better and better.'
- Say to yourself 'It is easy – and I can.'

It is impossible to think of two different things at the same time; if we say something, then that is the only thought in our mind. So, to relieve pain say, rapidly and continuously so as to put all other thoughts out of your mind, 'It's going, going, going ... gone,' and, to reinforce the suggestion, gently massage the affected part. Say it with faith and leave the unconscious to do its work. To make suggestions acceptable to the subconscious they must be made without effort. The subconscious has a marvellous memory, accepts what it is told and is responsible for the functioning of all our organs, by the intermediary of our brain.

- 'The will must not be brought into play in practising autosuggestion. The will always yields to the imagination – this is an absolute rule which admits of no exceptions.'
- 'Every thought entirely filling our mind becomes true for us and tends to transform itself into action.'
- 'Autosuggestion is the influence of the imagination upon the moral and physical being of mankind.'

It is necessary to train the imagination and then build up self-confidence, based on actual evidence of the power of the imagination. If you lack confidence in your powers at first, this will give place to self-confidence when based on the knowledge of what this force can do, as evidenced by results of only a short time in practising the method.

As the unconscious is the 'director' of all our functions we can therefore – through the subconscious – order a malfunctioning organ to perform properly. We possess within us a force of incalculable power. If we direct it in a conscious and wise manner it gives us the mastery of ourselves, and makes it possible to help others to escape from physical and mental ills.

The subconscious supervises body functions. One can stop haemorrhages, cure constipation, migraine, ulcers, etc., using autosuggestion to make the organs function normally again.

When making conscious autosuggestions make them without any effort, i.e. without using the will. Be sure (i.e. believe) that you will obtain what you want – and you will obtain it. To become master of oneself it is enough to think that one is becoming so. We can be what we make ourselves, and not what circumstances make us.

Fear is the most destructive autosuggestion. Fear is surrounded by an aura of emotion which considerably intensifies its effect. One must have optimism always, and in spite of everything, even when events do not seem to justify it. 'Every idea which exclusively occupies the mind is transformed into an actual physical or mental state.' The efforts we make to conquer an idea by exerting the will only serve to make that idea more powerful.

An organic disease may be increased a hundredfold by allowing the mind to brood on it. Even in the most serious organic diseases the element contributed by wrong thought is infinitely greater than that which is purely physical. Whatever thought we continually think, if it is reasonable, tends to become an actual condition of our life.

Leave the subconscious to bring about the right conditions in its own way. Only the desired end result must be thought about and suggested to the subconscious. The body wisdom knows best.

Never exert any effort in making suggestions. Efforts made to conquer an idea, through the use of the will (e.g. the idea of pain, etc.), will only serve to make that idea more powerful.

The practice of autosuggestion is one that is readily available to everyone, but it does require a lot of concentration. The benefits, however, are incalculable.

FURTHER READING

The quotes in this chapter are from Emile Coue, taken from the books *Self Mastery Through Conscious Autosuggestion* by Emile Coue and *The Practice of Autosuggestion by the Method of Emile Coue* by C. Harry Brooks.

31
IMAGERY AND VISUALISATION

Following on from the ideas of Coue, in which, as we have seen, positive suggestions are given to the mind, techniques have also been developed involving relaxation and mentally imagining any desired state of health. The imagination is a very powerful force, for good or ill. It is fairly obvious that worries or persistent negative emotions (the basis on which cures through the Bach flower remedies are based) can initiate a chain reaction of symptoms of ill health, such as headaches, insomnia, stomach ulcers, heart palpitations. It is not so obvious, but equally true, that mental activity can initiate a healing process too.

The body's immune system is in indirect contact with and is influenced by the mind; our thinking and emotions can therefore have actual physical repercussions on the lymphocyte population which is the first line of the body's defence system. The mind can thus be used prophylactically to prevent disease from appearing, and therapeutically to help the body heal itself. This has been shown by the new science called psychoneuroimmunology (PNI), which has shown conclusively the link between the mind and the lymphocytes.

To influence the mind there are several comparatively simple techniques which require complete relaxation in order to visualise the state desired. Once this relaxation state is attained there then needs to be some form of guided imagery or visualisation of the state of health desired. Relaxation of itself can actually help activate one's bodily defences, but directed imagery, which is really a visual result of auto-suggestion as propounded by Emile Coue, has even more impact on the feelings and emotions which are so important in influencing the physical responses to stresses of all kinds.

The aim of visualisation is to imagine health in the minutest detail, all the time believing it is possible to reach a state of health. Autosuggestive techniques, as outlined in the previous chapter, are in themselves effective, but imagery, which works through mental 'parables', impresses the desired end even more strongly on the mind and therefore has a greater effect on those physical processes which are protective and strengthening.

RELAXATION

First it is necessary to get into a state of 'near' sleep, the sort of condition one is in when just dropping off to sleep. Sit comfortably with a straight back, feet on the ground (if you lie down you are likely to go off to sleep completely), with your eyes closed. There should not be any confusing sounds around which would misdirect your attention; many people, though, do find that soothing music, perhaps of birdsong, the sound of the sea, etc., helps to get one into the right kind of mood to distance oneself from everyday happenings. The Silva method of mind control uses the technique of looking upwards, under closed lids, and this, after a little practice, can bring you into the 'alpha' state, the state of being half awake and half asleep.

If you feel your mind wandering, concentrate on the separate parts of the body, starting with the feet and working upwards. Consciously relax your toes, ankles, calves, knees, thigh muscles, and so on up the body. We are often unaware of the tension that we habitually carry in some muscles. While relaxing, the fears and thoughts of one's ailment temporarily disappear and make it more possible to think positively about a happy outcome to the illness.

VISUALISATION

Now concentrate on what you want – which is obviously relief from pain and full health. There is really no benefit to be gained from saying to oneself 'I have no pain' when obviously there is pain. On the other hand, it is of value to visualise yourself as completely healthy and without pain, doing the things you want to do. As you gain confidence the feeling of hopelessness will disappear, which will in its turn give you more confidence – a helpful rather than a vicious circle.

The more you can relax, the more concentration you can give to these worthy objectives. As Coue said, think of a desired occurrence, believe that it will happen, and it will. The more you manage to concentrate the mind, the more you will believe in its power to have a physical effect on the body.

Visualisation or mental imagery is not for everyone. However, some people find it beneficial to think of cancer cells as being invading armies, or unpleasant organisms that need wiping out. Personally, being of a rather logical way of thinking, I would prefer to think of them as normal cells which have been contaminated and need destroying by the macrophages which I can imagine as larger bodies with engulfing arms. If I envisage them as coming in overwhelming numbers then victory is assured. Always imagine victory for the 'goodies' over the 'baddies'. Visualisation is most effective when one knows the processes of the body and can accurately 'see' the desired processes working. There must be a clear mental picture of what needs to be done. The mind has to give 'instructions' to the body, and this is only possible if there is adequate knowledge of these processes.

Visualisation is the link between the conscious and the subconscious autonomic mind which actually instructs the body to carry out its operations; this autonomic mind must therefore be contacted and instructed before any physical results can happen. The more specific a mental command is, the more likely it is to be carried out. No effort can be involved in making these instructions.

The will must not be brought into the visualisation. Using one's will implies a possibility of losing, i.e. the imagination will be telling you there is a possibility that you will not be able to bring about the condition you want. And here there is no apology for repeating Coue's words: 'Where the will and the imagination are in conflict, the imagination always wins.' Visualise all the time that the desired progress has already started. In the words of Al Koran in *Bring Out the Magic in your Mind* (Tandem), 'Images are the language of the subconscious.'

32
CARING

Medicine has become technologically oriented. Often there is not enough time, or adequate staff, to carry out integrated care in the home. It is a primary aim of places like the Cancer Centre at Springhill to extend the quality of care and to show the influence that family and friends have in caring. Hospitals tend to take over all control; but while providing the best nursing care, they can often disregard the feelings and intentions of the families and others who care. Hospitals are, happily, just coming round to including relatives and friends in their caring service.

The hospice movement, with its outstanding ability to provide care in conjunction with members of the family, is primarily for providing the best quality of life at its end. Springhill is best suited for intermediate care and education, and to give strength and comfort in a home from home atmosphere; it is a place where people are given time to think and a time to change.

A deep void inevitably opens when someone on the hospital staff says in a detached way, 'There is nothing more that can be done for you here. Go home until things get so bad that you have to return.' There is a natural horror at such a statement, a paralysing fear when one is told one is incurable. There is, however, much that can be done, both by increasing the quality of life and in helping towards long-term remission of the disease. Caring establishments like Springhill are not there to replace the NHS, but they can provide a more humane extension of care, encompassing relatives and friends as part of the caring team.

Potential carers should be prepared to ask themselves some questions:

- Does the patient really want care? The answer may be obvious, but some people resent being helpless patients and do not like excessive sympathy.
- As a carer do I, can I, really care?
- Does the patient want to be touched?
- Can I, as a carer, bear to touch the patient in his/her present state?
- Is the patient frightened?
- How do I react as a carer? Frightened too? There are questions,

pain, totally new situations and responsibilities to face. Deep down carers are often frightened, although this fear is not often acknowledged.

There then grows a commitment between the carer and the patient. An ability develops, often on both sides, to read the messages coming from each individual. Carers may then go beyond duty, or any pre-established concepts of care, so that a new relationship is engendered.

Holistic caring is all about the growth of relationships, healing relationships, and unfolding the potential for every relationship to be a healing one. This will be regardless of the fact that the person, the patient, may not live, may not be healed in the physical sense; yet spiritually they may be healed and ready to pass, in peace, on to their next phase, the realm of the spirit life. It is therefore important to help people express themselves emotionally in a way that perhaps they could not manage at home or in a hospital situation.

Holistic care is very much about helping patients to take some responsibility for their own health, physically and mentally. The orthodox approach is primarily to intervene and take over, instead of building on what is already there – the family and friends, and the patient's responsibility for his own health. The technological side has to be kept within bounds, be more compassionate, conciliatory and less interventionist.

Caring should not completely take over the patient's sense of self-care and self-responsibility until the patient is beyond caring for himself. It is the duty of carers to help and not obstruct the unfolding of a sense of self-care, self-responsibility, both on the part of the patient and the relatives and friends. It is tremendously important, when a crisis approaches, for relatives and friends to be actively involved.

33
DYING WITH DIGNITY

We are only people in transit on our life's journey. When death has to be faced there are bound to be fears, uncertainty, sorrows, but death is nothing less than the promise of eternal life. The fear of the unknown is the main fear of the patient. Some people want to go, to be free, and they should be allowed to go, to give up the struggle in dignity and peace; people who have died and been brought back say it was a most wonderful experience.

When the fear of death is reduced, physical pain is also reduced – an acknowledgment that one is dying reduces fear. In doing so one should review what goals one can still aim for in order to obtain peace of mind. If you have cancer or have to face the possibility of dying, it may prove fruitful to consider:

- Your mental reactions to a recurrence of your disease, i.e. is it a prelude to death or only a temporary setback?
- Have you a particular image of how you will die?
- How do you think your family and friends will react to your death?
- What happens to your consciousness after death?
- What have you done with your life?
- What resentments do you still harbour?
- What would you do if you had your life over again?

Appreciate that even a change in feelings is a kind of death and rebirth process, a process of creating positive new attitudes, a process in which you allow yourself to become more the type of person you would like to be.

Care of the dying should be aimed at helping a person to be ready to go when the time is right, instead of trying to block the natural process. The whole subject should be discussed with the patient. One should be very wary of intervening; death should be a liberating process and we should all know when to stop providing more than palliative care. Many carers tend not to allow the natural spontaneous transition from life to death. Hospices are places which allow this process to take place with the least amount of discomfort and, more importantly, free of fear and, as far as possible, free of pain.

There has developed a certain arrogance as to what has to be done when terminally ill people are in great pain. Specialist nurses are often very incisive about pain control, maintaining that it should be carried out in this or that way. It is important to dispel a lot of the mystique of pain control; there is a reason for the pain, which has a life cycle of its own.

When one is caring for someone who is preparing for death, physically and mentally, it is important to lessen their physical burden, if possible, and make sure their organs are not overloaded. It is not helpful to give big meals, or the patient will become more and more putrid, with the distressing smell of death increasing. Give very light foods that are easily digested. The more the body is involved in trying to break down difficult foods, the longer it will hold on. The cleaner the body is, the easier and more natural dying is: the heavier it is with decaying matter, the longer it takes to die and the more pain there will be.

There should be more education or counselling on many aspects of the dying process and its natural place in the scheme of things, particularly for relatives, who are often woefully ignorant of such matters. They should be made aware of the fact that the patient has nothing to be afraid of. It is the relatives who have fears – perhaps a fear of being left alone, a fear of having to do without the support of a strong member of the family, a fear of the responsibility of having to cope with a dying person – and they feel that, naturally, hospitals have the necessary equipment and expertise to handle any crisis. Relatives may find hard to accept any suggestion that they should have classes to learn the arts of caring, but subsequently they could realise how helpful they have been.

At the end of a life, we all need counselling. Or, looked at from another angle, we are all counsellors and carers when we are in contact with a terminally ill person, whatever job we do; especially as it is probably a situation that has been forced on us without our being able to prepare for it. We all need direction and information.

From the patient's point of view, each person needs individual handling. What one person can enjoy may be anathema to another. Noise levels in particular should be monitored carefully. Perhaps, one, or at most two, visitors at a time can be coped with. There must be peace and tranquillity above all else. Dying should be treated as a sacred episode. Furthermore, given the right atmosphere, the carers themselves will not feel so drained.

There are of course many families and friends very actively concerned with the care of loved ones who are dying; they do not leave the burden entirely in the hands of the professionals. And the situation is now being ameliorated by hospice care, which has brought a lot of humanity to dying. Furthermore, nurses are now being taught that the patient's happiness and peace of mind are all that matters, although their schedule of work often does not leave them the time to follow this excellent precept.

Carers, whether they are relatives, friends or hospice workers, represent what the *Lancet* called the fourth state of medicine, the many voluntary groups and individuals in the community available to provide whatever back-up is required. Their presence should never be underestimated. They are a very dedicated army of people, with a commitment that makes the atmosphere and manner of caring so outstanding. They give so much, particularly in a quality of care that many in the professions cannot provide due to the pressures of time and of their many commitments. For example, only about 15 per cent of the helpers at Springhill are salaried, all the rest being devoted part- or full-time voluntary carers; and this devotion is reflected in the caring attitude found at all levels at Springhill.

Appendixes

AMINO ACIDS AND PROTEINS

Amino acids are the building blocks of proteins, each protein being made up of different numbers, combinations and arrangements of amino acids. Proteins are the sum of a number of amino acids, and the manner in which they are put together determines the protein's role in the body. Put simply, the nature of a protein is determined by:

- The sequence in which the amino acids are linked.
- The amounts of each amino acid.

Proteins fulfil many roles in the human body and may be:

- Enzymes, made from amino acids, together with vitamins as cofactors and minerals as activators.
- Hormones, which travel round the body to exert their influence on cells in another area.
- Oxygen carriers.

Two amino acids linked together make a peptide (e.g. enkephaline pain killers), three amino acids linked together make a tripeptide, and more than three amino acids make a polypeptide (e.g. hair, muscle fibres). If the polypeptide is folded in a three-dimensional structure it forms proteins such as haemoglobin, insulin, albumen, globulins.

When proteins are eaten, they are broken down by digestive juices into amino acids and most are absorbed by the bloodstream, transported to the tissues and then recombined into different proteins, although some remain as 'free' amino acids. For example, some amino acids are made into enzymes; therefore any shortage may mean the body will be unable to make proper use of the proteins eaten. Others will go into nails, blood cells, brain cells, etc., while others may go into glands which manufacture hormones which help break down and build up human proteins.

Digestive enzymes in gastric juices, followed by enzymes from the pancreas and the bile in the small intestine, work on protein in food, breaking it down into amino acids, which are then absorbed and go to the liver for processing and distribution. If there are insufficient digestive enzymes, the proteins we eat will not be broken down completely and will therefore putrefy in the small intestine, producing toxic byproducts which may in turn give rise to food allergies, mental and emotional disturbances, rheumatism, arthritis, gout, etc. It may then be necessary to supplement the diet with digestive enzymes to ensure better protein breakdown.

Digestion of proteins in the stomach must be done in an acid medium, so taking bicarbonate of soda, which neutralises the acid in the stomach, will result in proteins we have eaten not being adequately digested. People with diarrhoea do not digest protein properly and therefore some will be wasted.

DNA and RNA (which are in every cell) organise amino acids, through a genetic coding, into particular protein molecules. If the DNA and/or RNA is damaged, then the resultant protein may not be correctly formed and the body's defence system will reject them, as it would any foreign proteins, bacteria or viruses. Certain amino acids are required for the repair of DNA and RNA.

Amino acids are thus required in a particular relationship to produce certain chemicals in the body, i.e. they are precursors to these chemicals. Therefore any alteration, excess or shortage, in the supply of amino acids is likely to affect the chemicals produced, leading to various ailments. For instance, any alteration in the proportions of amino acids making up the neurotransmitters serotonin, dopamine or noradrenaline will result in behavioural disorders, neurotransmitters being chemicals which carry messages from one nerve to another or from a nerve to a target tissue.

All cells extract amino acids from the bloodstream and assemble them into the particular growth requirements of the cell involved. Fast growing malignant cells have an abnormally high need for and an accumulation of free amino acids, significantly higher than those in the surrounding normal tissue. Proteins cannot be manufactured if an essential amino acid is missing; therefore if a malignant tumour can be deprived of an essential amino acid, reproduction of the cell cannot go on. For example it has been found that a phenylalanine-free diet helps to reduce tumour activity.

Some amino acids compete with others for transport round the body and also compete at particular sites in the body. Therefore an excess or deficiency of one amino acid may hinder, for better or worse, the effectiveness of another. If any of the particular amino acids (or minerals or vitamins) are absent, cell function will be slowed and therefore will age more quickly. The more proteins are eaten, the more vitamin B6 and magnesium is required for use in metabolising them; these are essential, together with vitamin C, for the assimilation of amino acids in the body.

The relative quantities of amino acids in any particular food determines its nutritional value. Therefore combining foods with different levels of amino acids can produce a complete protein meal, e.g. wheat products are deficient in lysine, whereas legumes have more than enough. (This should not be confused with the Hay system, which specifies what foods should be combined with each other purely for the purpose of not mixing proteins and carbohydrates for digestive purposes – see Chapter 24.)

Proteins are found mainly in:

- Milk, liver, kidneys and eggs, which are the best sources of complete proteins.
- Meat, fish.
- Nuts, soybeans, wheatgerm, vegetables, grains.

Foods which contain proteins with amino acid ratios that closely resemble those of the body are called high-quality protein; for example, on a scale of 1–100, breastmilk rates as 100, whole eggs as 94, cows' milk as 85, meat, poultry, fish as 76–86, rice as 80 and potatoes as 78. Some foods have a preponderance of one amino acid and high-quality protein can be obtained by combining these foods.

Essential amino acids are not manufactured by the body and must be obtained through the diet; they are isoleucine, leucine, lysine, methionine, phenylalanine, threonine, tryptophan, valine.

Amino acids which require essential amino acids for their production are cystine and taurine, which are made from methionine, and tyrosine, which is made from phenylalanine.

Non-essential amino acids – which are actually still essential for protein production but which are manufactured by the body in normally sufficient quantities – are arginine, alanine, aspartic acid, cysteine, cystine, glutamic acid, glycine, histidine, hydroxyproline, proline, serine, taurine, tyrosine.

Some non-essential amino acids can be looked on as contingency amino acids, which may become essential; for instance arginine, which is normally produced by the body, may not be produced in sufficient amounts in young people. A body's requirement for a particular amino acid can easily outstrip its ability to produce enough, particularly in both the young and the elderly.

Semi-essential amino acids are those necessary for normal growth and development, but which are not required for maintenance of our nitrogen balance.

Deficiencies of amino acids mean:

- The body will be unable to make proper use of proteins eaten;

digestion will be poor, resulting in a shortage of amino acids derived from the protein, i.e. a kind of chain reaction.

- Inefficient breakdown of proteins means putrefaction in the small intestine, resulting in gas and toxins. This happens particularly in people over 35 to 40 who may need to supplement their diet with digestive enzymes (plus betaine hydrochloride, as after the age of 40 people do not generally secrete sufficient hydrochloric acid).

Since amino acids are used by the body to form the proteins it requires, in the form it can use, supplementation saves the necessary step of breaking down dietary protein into these amino acids. But when considering the use of individual amino acid supplements, note that the manufacture of the final chemical also involves vitamins and minerals too. Also note that individual requirements can be highly variable.

ENZYMES AND COENZYMES

Enzymes are made from amino acids and are present in every living cell of man and plants. They are catalysts only, i.e. they bring about a chemical change, but without being involved in the change themselves. Furthermore they are specific, each being for a different purpose, a different reaction. Many enzymes consist of two parts – a protein part (i.e. the amino acids) and a cofactor portion (made up of vitamins or mineral ions). This latter portion is normally called the coenzyme.

- Cold inactivates enzymes, and they remain dormant.
- Heat above 104°F denatures many mammalian enzymes.
- The acidity or alkalinity is important; pepsin, an enzyme which breaks down protein in the stomach, likes an acid pH of 1.2 to 1.8, while trypsin, an enzyme from the pancreas, likes an alkaline pH of about 8.2.

Enzymes must be continually replaced, as one operation may destroy an enzyme; e.g. digestive enzymes are destroyed by the changes of pH as they pass along the digestive tract.

The best sources of food from which enzymes are made are vegetables, fruit, nuts and seeds. If more raw food is eaten the body will not have to work so hard to manufacture more enzymes. It is useful to eat a raw salad before a cooked meal to protect the enzymes which will help digestion. The ideal to aim at is 60 per cent raw food. Some enzymes in the brassica family combine with iodine and prevent it reaching the thyroid; therefore it is useful to take 1 tsp kelp daily. Canned foods have had their enzymes destroyed by heating.

Enzymes are generally named after the chemical which is to be changed, e.g. phosphatase helps the chemical change of phosphorus, sucrase helps the chemical change of sucrose.

Antioxidant enzymes are produced by the body and remove cell-damaging free radicals. These important enzymes include:

- Superoxide dismutase (or SOD) – removes the superoxide radical.
- Glutathione peroxidase (which includes selenium) – removes both lipid peroxide and hydrogen peroxide.

- Catalase – removes hydrogen peroxide. Catalase is the primary enzyme involved in the immune system. The best sources of catalase are, in foods eaten raw:
  - onion, carrot, sweet potato, sweet pepper, garlic.
  - banana, tomato, pear, apple, maize, melon, orange, lemon.
  - egg yolks, whole wheat, cheese, liver.

  Note that catalase is naturally synthesised in the body in response to stress, sufficient only to ensure normal response to things like cold, anxiety, etc. Daily exercise is sufficient to provide the necessary stress of a natural kind to initiate catalase production.
- Hyaluronidase – an enzyme secreted by cancerous tumour cells that dissolves collagen. To inactivate hyaluronidase and to strengthen collagen, give megadoses of vitamin C.
- Methione reductase – removes the hydroxyl radical.
- Coenzyme Q10 – protects against lipid peroxides.

COENZYME Q10

Quinone is a coenzyme. Its name forms part of the word ubiquinone (ubiquitous quinone = found in every cell), which is another name for coenzyme Q. Coenzyme Q10 (the only one found in man) is essential for the production of cellular energy, which in turn is responsible for all energy requirements of the body, particularly in the construction and reconstruction of cells which are constantly dying and being replaced. CoQ10 is a fat-soluble substance, which can now be produced artificially by fermentation and extraction from microorganisms. The best natural source of CoQ10 is beef muscle and heart.

CoQ is found in all living plants and animals, but there are various types, depending on the number of side chains of oxygen, hydrogen and carbon. Only CoQ10 (i.e. with a side chain of ten groups of five atoms) is useful to humans, but other formations, e.g. CoQ9, CoQ8, etc., can be converted by the body to form CoQ10, although this ability is reduced as we get older, leading to a CoQ10 deficiency in middle and old age and leaving the body less able to fight middle age diseases such as heart disease or cancer.

No side effects have been noted in the use of CoQ10. It is useful as a protective 'buffer' to reduce possible side effects of a therapeutic drug.

Cells convert nutrients they receive from the diet into an energy-storage molecule, adenosine triphosphate (ATP), and the energy is then released as and when required, for all energy-requiring processes in the cell. The amount of ATP in the body at any one time is very small (about three ounces in all) and therefore it must be topped up constantly from the foods eaten and stored, which are then converted by coenzyme Q10 into ATP. This coenzyme is therefore extremely important in the production of energy for all systems in the body.

The immune system is crucially important in the way a person responds to illness and stress and obviously requires a lot of energy to keep it going. As coenzyme Q10 is a key function in the energy-producing process, it follows that keeping up levels of this coenzyme in the body will help the immune system – it increases the utilisation of energy available to every cell in the immune system. For example, CoQ10 increases production of the antibody IgG (which coats microorganisms to make them more palatable and speed their uptake by the scavenger immune cells); these increases of antibodies have bolstered the immune defences in cancers of the breast and lung, in cardiac failure and in diabetes. CoQ10 is also a powerful antioxidant, although supplementation may have to be for at least eight weeks before there is likely to be a noticeable response.

Vitamin E boosts the body's synthesis of CoQ10 and this may be one reason why vitamin E is useful in boosting the immune system. Selenium too is required in the production of CoQ10 and, through this, increases its use as a anti-cancer agent. There are no adverse reactions, but as it has not been tested on pregnant or lactating females it should not be used on such patients yet.

Coenzyme Q10 has been found useful in many kinds of heart problems, although a proportion of heart complaints will of course stem from causes other than a shortage of CoQ10.

- Diseased hearts have very significant CoQ10 deficiencies, and in fact may be diseased as a result of this deficiency.
- Beta blockers inhibit enzymes that are dependent on CoQ10, supplementation of which may ensure sufficient of these enzymes are available. It may also help prevent other common side effects of beta blockers.
- CoQ10 will offset the adverse immunosuppressive effects on the heart of chemotherapy drugs such as Cytoxan or Adriamycin, but does not adversely affect their anti-tumour activity.
- Exercise is the best means of strengthening the heart (and incidentally increases CoQ in the heart tissues), but if this is not possible then supplementation with CoQ10 will improve heart function even at rest, as if exercise had been undertaken. As CoQ10 levels in the heart will drop after a few weeks if supplementation is stopped, it is prudent to keep on with a maintenance dose for as long as necessary (no adverse effects of long-term usage have been recorded).

- CoQ10 has been found useful in protecting patients who have major heart surgery, e.g. cardiac valve replacements or bypass operations, or organ transplants, or who have suffered brain damage as a result of an accident.
- The myocardium (muscular inner layer of the heart) is protected by CoQ10.
- Infarct size as a result of a coronary occlusion is reduced by CoQ10.
- The frequency of angina attacks is reduced by CoQ10.
- CoQ10 may be able to reduce the amount of cardiac drugs such as digitalis that have to be taken (thereby reducing the normal risks of overdosage and side effects of digitalis therapy).
- Congestive heart failure, induced by overstimulation of the thyroid gland, may be because of a shortage of CoQ10.
- Irregular heart beats (arrhythmias) as a result of hypoxia (lack of oxygen to the tissues and consequent increase in toxic chemicals in the tissues) have been experimentally normalised through supplementation with CoQ10.
- Patients with high blood pressure (hypertension) often show a deficiency of CoQ10 and supplementation reduces the need for diuretics or anti-hypertensive drugs.
- Electrical impulses regulating the heartbeat may become blocked, causing irregular beats; CoQ10 has been found to restore the normal rhythm.
- Through obvious improvement in oxygen utilisation as a result of CoQ10 supplementation in heart diseases, without additional exercise, patients feel a new will to live and there is an obvious improvement in their mental well-being.

Most people show a deficiency of CoQ10 as they grow older and are therefore likely to show a beneficial response quickly to supplementation. Fewer tumours will develop and those that do have been found to be significantly smaller when adequate CoQ10 is taken.

CoQ10 boosts chemotherapy or hydrocortisone treatment of leukaemia and helps to reduce the drugs' side effects; by boosting their effectiveness, it can reduce the quantity of drugs given. Note that cortisone is an immunosuppressive drug, so CoQ10, which helps the immune system, will counteract the bad effect of cortisone. The effectiveness of vitamin E and selenium as anti-cancer agents is probably linked to their ability to boost CoQ10 biosynthesis, thus helping the immune system. It has been suggested that CoQ10 should be designated a vitamin. But vitamins have to be converted in the body to coenzymes, so CoQ10 is one stage further on as it is already a coenzyme.

The benefits of CoQ10 supplementation will be greater if a person has an obvious deficiency, and it may take some weeks before benefits are felt. It does however have immediate effect when used as a protective 'buffer' to reduce possible side effects when taking a drug. Dosages of 90 mg per day of CoQ10 may be necessary (and safe) for pathological heart muscle problems, although for chronic angina a dosage of 150 mg per day has been found necessary. Dosages will in general be directly proportional to the severity of the disease being treated. Mild diseases show only a small deficiency of CoQ10, while the deficiency increases with the severity of the disease and the dosage required may reach 100 to 150 mg per day in advanced cases of heart failure.

VITAMIN C

Vitamin C (ascorbic acid) is known as the 'anti-stress' vitamin. It is a carbohydrate, produced from glucose, by the action of enzymes, and is present in nearly all plants and animals – apart from man, guinea pigs and some monkeys. In plants, seeds have no ascorbic acid, but as soon as the plant embryo starts to develop, ascorbic acid is immediately formed. This is why sprouted seeds are a good source of this vitamin.

It is an extraordinarily useful vitamin, as can be seen from the following list:

- It is the prime antioxidant. It protects against lipid peroxidation and is a free radical scavenger. It works very much faster as an antioxidant than other antioxidants like selenium. It penetrates the interstitial fluid round the cells and stops the oxidation process, allowing time for cell repair. It is also a carrier for antioxidant particles from other areas to the damaged area. It is not an anti-cancer agent, nor a direct anti-tumour factor, but, being a major antioxidant, it can inhibit the activity of malignant cells and the deterioration of cells that have been wounded.
- It is antiviral, capable of inactivating and destroying viruses such as those of polio, herpes, foot and mouth, rabies, hepatitis, the common cold and flu.
- It is antiseptic.
- It is antibacterial and will inactivate toxic bacteria responsible for diphtheria, tetanus, dysentery. It may of course kill good bacteria if used in very high doses, so when using it as an antioxidant against food deterioration it is better to spray the food only with a low dose.
- It increases the activity of macrophages (part of the body's defence system of phagocytes). This helps protect against infectious diseases by assisting the process of phagocytosis, by which white cells engulf and digest bacteria – this process is directly related to the ascorbic acid content of blood.
- It stimulates the production of T-killer cells which are called on to attack viruses that have infected any body cells. It thus stimulates the immune system, which is the body's defence system.
- It helps the liver to fight infection.
- It improves enzyme activity.
- It helps keep down cholesterol levels and is therefore useful in preventing heart troubles.

- It strengthens and helps to form collagen (which is about one-third of the body's protein), so is useful in the continual process of self-repair and self-maintenance of the tissues. It has been found that cancer tumour cells produce an enzyme hyaluronidase which dissolves collagen; therefore strengthening the collagen with 10 grams daily of vitamin C will help counter the effect of this enzyme.
- It counters the ill-effects of drugs which drastically reduce the amount of vitamin C in the blood.
- It accelerates the rate of natural cortisone production by the adrenal glands.
- It helps prevent the conversion of nitrites (already converted from nitrates) into nitrosamines, which are cancerous.
- It is useful in preventing colds – take a little every hour or half hour. This gets rid of the catarrh and no more should be formed.
- Similarly when bloating or gassy, take a little often to repair cell material very quickly.
- It helps sore throats, tonsillitis, tooth decay, cataracts, muscles and cartilages (easy bruising indicates there is probably a shortage of vitamin C).
- It prevents strokes, heart disease, atherosclerosis (hardening of the arteries) and keeps arteries open in general.
- It decreases pain in arthritis and multiple sclerosis.
- Shortage produces scurvy or scurvy-type symptoms.
- Being water soluble it protects the bladder from cancer.
- It counters biochemical stresses, bacterial and viral infections, and stresses of all kinds, but in particular those due to chemotherapy or surgery (useful to take before operations and post-operatively to assist healing).
- Helps to carry fluorides out of the system, thus counteracting the ill effects of the fluoridation of water.
- Helpful in leukaemia through strengthening of collagen and tissues.
- Has a beneficial effect on secondary bone cancers (at least 10 grams a day is required).
- Helps against cancers caused by ultra-violet rays and certain chemical pollutants such as benzopyrene.
- It is a natural antihistamine.
- It is a non-toxic diuretic in large doses.

VITAMIN C AND CANCER

- Vitamin C reduces the pains of cancer.
- The recurrence of bladder cancer, due to smoking, etc., can be prevented by large doses daily.
- The effects of toxic drugs given in treatment can be offset by large doses. However, Linus Pauling clearly stated that 'vitamin C therapy is almost entirely vitiated if the patient has previously been subjected to chemotherapy or radiation'. Vitamin C therapy should therefore be administered before chemotherapy if possible.
- The degree of malignancy is determined inversely by the degree of connective tissue resistance, which in itself is dependent on the adequacy of ascorbic acid level in the body.
- In leukaemics it has been found that there are considerable shortages of ascorbic acid, mostly locked in by excessive white cells, when tissues become weak and collagen production stops.

VITAMIN C LOSS

Vitamin C in the body can be lost through prolonged treatment with ACTH, or cortisone, antibiotics or sulfa drugs. It is also lost through exposure to environmental toxins, car fumes, smoking, and prolonged exposure to light and heat. Most cooking causes a loss of the vitamin from food. People under stress use it up quicker than healthy people.

Deficiencies may cause gastric and intestinal disorders, loss of calcium and phosphorus from bones, tooth decay, a tendency to haemorrhages and poor healing of wounds, bleeding gums, weight loss, shortness of breath, rapid respiration and heartbeat, anaemia, atrophy of glands and organs, joint pains. The first signs of deficiency may be bruising, nosebleeds and bleeding gums.

TAKING VITAMIN C

A small number of people may be hypersensitive to vitamin C so start with low doses. Reactions may include sickness, depression, gastric distress, vomiting, diarrhoea, headache, skin rashes, all of which disappear on reducing the dosage for a while. Also women on the contraceptive pill should not normally take more than 1 g per day as this can intensify the effects of synthetic hormones. Megadoses of vitamin C may invalidate orthodox medical tests, so always advise your doctor of the quantity of vitamin C you are taking before having a test.

It is useful to know what level of vitamin C gives you diarrhoea (i.e.

your tolerance dose) so that you know what level you can go to in taking this vitamin to protect you against the side effects of chemotherapy.

Pure ascorbic acid is generally too acid, particularly for people with candida overgrowth. Ascorbic acid should therefore not be taken on its own. It is better to use ascorbic acid combined with calcium ascorbate which makes it more alkaline. It is best used with mineral water or one of the Breuss vegetable juices. Note that Redoxon has a certain level of sugar, plus pure ascorbic acid, thus increasing the level of acidity in the body. It is important to have vitamin C with liquid food from fresh plant material and the vitamin C gets carried along with it.

Soft fruits are very liable to fungal infestation, so wash them well or spray with a solution of vitamin C (about ¼ tsp to ½ pint of water) to stop oxidation (or one can use another antioxidant like a lemon). It is useful to have a spray of vitamin C handy in the kitchen to spray any vegetable or fruit that is cut, to stop oxidation. Vegetables sprayed with vitamin C retain a better cellular structure and do not disintegrate.

When eating fruit always have vitamin C with it. If you find that a particular food is likely to upset you, take a gram of vitamin C before or after the meal.

Soak any nuts, seeds, pulses and beans in vitamin C overnight and they become enzyme-rich again, although it may take a couple of days to get cereals, corn and beans to become 'live' again. Vitamin C, being a fungicide and bactericide, helps to block the activity of any fungus or toxin.

VITAMIN C FLUSH

If you have candidiasis or cancer, it is good to take occasional vitamin C flushes because the whole of the intestines, and perhaps even the stomach, the oesophagus, larynx, the trachea, etc. are probably full of systemic fibroids. If the gut wall is entirely coated with a thick layer of mucus, fungal fibroids and noxious bacteria like *E. coli*, the nutrients will not be absorbed from the food; instead food which has not been broken down will be excreted, without absorption taking place into the bloodstream. That is why cancer patients often lose weight, as the body is living on the reservoir of nutrients that have been stored in it. Flushing out the system with vitamin C is the most successful way of eliminating toxins. It is quite amazing how pain is greatly relieved when there is a flushing out of toxins.

It is important to use completely dissolvable vitamin C powder. Take 2 grams every 15 minutes in a little juice – do not take too much water at this time. Continue until you reach bowel tolerance (when you may have as many as 20 bowel movements), which may not be until you have had 30 grams or more. It is important not to eat during the flush.

If you are very constipated it may be necessary also to take 2 tsps of Epsom salts and 2 tsps of olive oil to lubricate the liver, on which it works specifically. Alternate the vitamin C with the Epsom salts and olive oil.

THE ALIMENTARY OR DIGESTIVE SYSTEM

When food enters the mouth it is worked on physically by chewing, and chemically by the alkaline saliva, of which as much as 2 pints might be produced in a day. The saliva comes from the three salivary glands, the parotid, sublingual and submandibular. These glands produce an enzyme ptyalin (or diastase), which starts the breakdown of starch, converting it into a sugar called maltose.

The action of mastication regulates the temperature of the food, cooling or warming it. The food is then swallowed and passes through the pharynx, down the oesophagus, which is about 25 cm long, and past the cardiac valve into the stomach.

The stomach has a number of different chemicals:

- Hydrochloric acid (HCl), which has the job of neutralising the alkaline salivary enzyme ptyalin so that the acid can work on the digestion of proteins.
- Pepsin, which is required to change proteins into soluble peptones, which are easily dissolved and can pass through membranes into the bloodstream.
- Rennin, the second gastric juice enzyme, needed to curdle milk products.
- A substance called 'the intrinsic blood building factor of Castle', which is necessary to absorb vitamin B12 in the small intestine. A deficiency of this intrinsic factor is a cause of anaemia.

In the stomach the food is turned into a creamy fluid called chyle, which is acid, and which leaves the stomach little by little through the pyloric valve, entering the duodenum, which is the first part of the small intestine (approximately 20–21 feet in total). Here the main enzyme digestion takes place. Into the duodenum bile from the liver and gall-bladder and sodium bicarbonate from the pancreas enter, both of which are alkaline. The acid of the chyle is thus neutralised and then made alkaline immediately it enters the duodenum.

The intestinal wall and pancreas have glands which produce enzymes:

- Erepsin, which breaks down peptones into amino acids, which build-up into flesh-forming protein.
- Invertase and maltase, which reduce sugars to glucose.
- Enterokinase, converting inactive trypsinogen from the pancreas into trypsin; trypsin also acts on proteins.

This food mass, now called chyme, passes through the rest of the small intestine, being 'massaged' along by the muscles in the intestinal walls, with the nutrients being gradually absorbed by means of the villi (small finger-like projections from the intestinal walls) and the action of intestinal bacteria, passing amino acids, glucose, salts and water-soluble vitamins via the hepatic portal vein into the bloodstream. Fats and fat-soluble vitamins A and D are meanwhile absorbed by the villi and passed into the lymph stream through the lacteal ducts.

Most of the nutrients are absorbed by the time the now mainly solid chyme passes from the small intestine through the ileocaecal valve into the colon, whose main function is the absorption of water into the bloodstream.

THE CIRCULATION SYSTEM

The circulation system has three objectives:

- To circulate the blood round the body and, in it, to carry oxygen from the lungs, essential nutrients from the alimentary canal, and hormones.
- To provide heat to the extremities.
- To remove waste products to the kidneys for excretion, and CO_2 to the lungs to be expired.

There are four subdivisions of the system:

- The coronary circulation, for supplying blood to the heart muscle itself. This is a 'closed circuit', used blood being returned to the heart.
- The systemic circulation, which takes the blood to every other part of the body, via the aorta, the arteries and then by various branches through arterioles and capillaries to the extremities, returning via the veins to the heart and a large vein called the vena cava.
- The pulmonary circulation, which again is a sort of closed circuit, in that 'used' blood in the heart needs to be oxygenated by being passed through the lungs. It is taken there by the pulmonary arteries and, after oxygenation, returns via the four pulmonary veins through the mitral valve into the heart.
- The portal circulation takes food products in the blood from the digestive organs (intestines and stomach) through the portal veins to the liver. Here a number of chemical actions and cleansing occur before the blood is returned, via the hepatic veins and through the inferior vena cava, to the heart.

BLOOD

Blood is a tissue in which cells float in liquid (plasma) and is made up of:

- Red cells (erythrocytes), formed in the bone marrow, whose job is to take up and transport oxygen. The oxygen combines with haemoglobin in the red cells; this is a crystalline protein material, containing iron, which is in the red blood corpuscles and gives the red colour to the blood. Simple haemoglobin is found in venous blood, but in the arteries there is oxyhaemoglobin, containing oxygen from the lungs. This gets broken down as the blood passes through the tissues, which take up the oxygen for their own use. In people with anaemia there is a marked deficiency of haemoglobin in the blood.

- White cells (leucocytes), which have a cleansing and scavenging job. White blood cells consist of B cells (produced in the bone marrow), which produce antibodies to help destroy invading viruses or bacteria, inactivate toxins and help remove dead or damaged tissue, and T cells (lymphocytes, produced in the lymph glands, spleen and thymus), which either help other immune system cells to do their job, or kill virus-infected cells.

Blood is a substance with many uses:

- It temporarily stores nutrients taken from food via the digestive tract.
- It transports nutrients and oxygen round the body.
- It transports waste materials.
- It circulates heat, primarily from the liver and muscles.
- It takes hormones from ductless glands to tissues that require them.
- It produces antibodies to deal with hostile germs and toxins.
- It can coagulate and so prevent haemorrhages.

Blood consists of about 48 per cent water, the rest solids, most of which are organic substances from the food eaten. The interstitial fluid is fluid flowing into the lymphatic vessels from the blood, less the white and red cells and large proteins, which are left in the capillaries.

THE LYMPHATIC
SYSTEM

The lymphatic system is for draining impurities out of the blood, for example toxins stored or produced in the blood. If the lymph gets very congested through impacted lymphatic nodules (glands), then there will generally be some cancer in the area of the body that is drained by that part of the lymph system.

The lymphatic system is really a system of tubes through which quite viscous thick fluid passes, its principal role being to carry protector lymphocytes that defend the body and have an important role in cleansing the blood. For instance if the lymph glands are raised, perhaps in the neck, armpit, groin, etc., then there will be illnesses such as cystitis, bronchitis, tonsillitis, etc. Lymphatic system disorders, after a long period of disturbances to the lymphatic system, often give rise to benign tumours or cysts or even cancers. If anyone has cancer of the lung, one knows that the lymphatic system, as well as the respiratory system, is involved; because the toxins will not have been shifted and will have backed up on the organs. This may affect speech, movement, gestures, moods, particularly if the blood/brain barrier is weak and allows toxins to get through, resulting in brain tissue degeneration.

Some people are born with a very congested lymphatic system and may not have a good enough immune system to shift the residual material in the lymph. They therefore develop, at a very early age, illnesses that are normally connected with old age, such as bone marrow cancer, severe muscular dystrophy, rheumatoid arthritis.

The lymphatic glands are part of the network of the lymphatic system that drains the interstitial fluid back into the blood; they act as filters, sweeping up toxic particles and microorganisms. Adenitis is inflammation of a gland; glands down the neck may become inflamed as a result of any infection of an area drained by the lymphatic system going to that gland, e.g. eczema on the head results in swollen glands behind the head or ears, a wound in the foot gives swollen inguinal glands in the groin.

Therapeutic aids to help circulation and the movement of fluids is best achieved by warmth of any kind, massage, and breathing exercises – the blood quickens and there is better lymphatic movement. When people have cancer they often feel either too hot or too cold, and never manage to get their temperature just right, because the circulation is affected (particularly in motor disorders).

Hodgkin's disease (or pseudo leukaemia or lymphadenoma) is the enlargement of the spleen and lymph glands in the neck, followed by glands in the armpits and the groin, producing anaemia, general languor, weakness and loss of weight. The spleen then swells and feels hard, the chest glands increase and press on the heart and lungs, resulting in a cough, breathlessness, pain and blueness of face. There may be intense itching and bronzing of skin. Finally there is emaciation and dropsy – all taking about six months. (Note: continual overstimulation of any gland will eventually lead to underfunctioning.)

Scrofula (or tuberculous glands) is common in children. It mainly affects glands in the neck, the chain of glands under the jaw and those running up the neck. They may become infected through the tonsils in the throat. The glands in the abdomen are then affected producing wasting called tabes mesenterica. The glands enlarge over several months, producing sinuses which go on discharging for years, finally healing with red puckered unsightly scars.

Glands on the left side of the neck are often prone to be diseased as a result of cancer of the digestive system. Glands in the armpit become affected early in cancer of the breast.

Herbal remedies for enlarged lymph glands are echinacea and St John's wort, while to help adjust glandular imbalances use *Agnus castus*, blue flag root.

THE ENDOCRINE SYSTEM

Vital life processes over which we have no control, such as normal growth, digestion, assimilation, production of energy, cardiac action, respiration, etc., depend in great measure upon the maintenance of a delicate equilibrium between the two divisions of the autonomic nervous system. This balance is markedly influenced by the internal secretions of the ductless glands – the endocrine glands – which act as governors over it. But the connection also works the other way; for example, emotions have a great influence on various bodily functions, with a reflex action on the glands through the nervous system, affecting also the pacemaker in the heart controlling heart rhythm.

Most constitutional afflictions are due to glandular dysfunction, and it is possible to trace like tendencies running through a family history (inherited miasms, as Hahnemann, founder of homoeopathy, called such tendencies). Whenever one has a malignant disease one should look at what the glands are doing as they are the 'master conductors' of any chemical or biochemical processes in the body.

Through our glands we are always adapting to the environment and to the conditions created through our diet and way of life. We are born with a 'blueprint' for our survival; if we acknowledge this fundamental pattern with which we have been endowed at birth, we restore conditions of good health. Usually we are fighting against our original pattern in a glandular and metabolic sense, being forced, through the circumstances of our lives, to operate against it.

All our glands are synergistic (intimately interconnected one with another). Whenever there is something happening which interrupts this intercommunication organised by the autonomic nervous system (the controller of glandular functions), this links up with the cerebellum, the seat of the unconscious, the seat of memory from the beginning of time. When we experience things like loneliness, guilt, fear, a lack of meaning in our lives, what is happening is that we are trying to deny that fear – we are in a state of shock and denial; the conscious midbrain, our thinking brain, is trying to deny that this is going to happen to us, we tense up our muscles, feet, hands, legs, neck muscles, etc., we enter into a state of fear. This can all be helped enormously by relaxation, either in a group or with one other person with whom one can build up trust and affection.

When we feel threatened in any way, or feel we can just explode, all the messages from the cerebellum to our glands and organs are interrupted because somewhere in the body – often in the neck area – there is a skeletal change; the shoulders are raised, the stomach is disturbed, adrenaline flows and tensions are locked in. Unless we are conscious of them, we cannot dissolve them. Relentlessly this process goes on, causing a constriction of capillaries, neurotransmitters, glands, organs, etc., so that the flow of blood and fluids is disturbed and swellings appear in some areas; there is a loss of muscle or flesh after only a few weeks, despite eating well. Possibly because fluids in the lymphatic system have become stagnant in certain areas the flow of fluids in that area is interrupted. For instance if a person has a breast off and the lymphatic ganglions are severed she will often get lymphoedema.

There is no communication between the cerebellum, the autonomous processes, the glands and the conscious plane. The consciousness may be initiating actions that are totally antagonistic to what is happening in the rest of the body, or commands are sent from the adrenals to respond to a state of alarm that does not really exist, when really the whole organism needs a totally different set of commands. In a panic-stricken individual, frightened to the core, the adrenals will send messages upwards to the thyroid and pituitary glands, totally in error.

It is therefore important to look at how our lives affect our glands, and a brief explanation of the principal endocrine glands may make this more apparent.

To begin with, hormones are chemical messengers which induce specific responses in distant target tissues (or other endocrine glands), i.e. they are catalysts and exercise chemical control over other organs. The endocrine glands are ductless glands, i.e. they are glands which do not release their chemicals directly into another organ but work by producing hormones which are released into the bloodstream which takes them to whatever part of the body they are required in. These hormones, by releasing chemical messengers, stimulate or suppress activities of certain cells in organs at a distance from the glands themselves.

The endocrine system affects all important functions of the body, including growth, reproduction, nutrition, protection and adaptation. It is therefore vitally important to the efficient working of the body.

THE PITUITARY

The pituitary (or hypophysis) is situated in the cavity of the sphenoid bone at the base of the skull. It has long been regarded as the master or supervisory gland, regulating the work of other glands, although recent work shows that the thymus may be more important.

The pituitary has two lobes:

- The anterior lobe is responsible for the production of hormones for regulating the thyroid, parathyroid, adrenals, pancreatic islets and mammary glands. One important hormone produced is ACTH, which increases the production of cortisone in the cortex of the adrenal gland. This lobe also regulates the growth of bones, cartilages and the secretion of milk.
- The posterior lobe (called the hypothalamus) produces hormones which help the kidneys to increase reabsorption of water, help the onset of labour in childbirth and stimulate the thyroid to produce thyroxin.

THE ADRENALS

The adrenals (or suprarenals, so called because there is one above and attached to each kidney) are made up of:

- The cortex (the outer part) which affects the gonads and also produces cortisone.
- The medulla (or inner part) which affects the sympathetic nervous system and produces adrenaline, the 'fight or flight' hormone which stimulates the liver to increase blood sugar, and nor-adrenaline which is distributed by and through the blood to many organs and tissues which need to take action in time of stress. The physical response is that the heart beats faster, voluntary muscles contract more strongly, carbohydrates stored in the muscles and liver are released into the bloodstream as a source of energy and blood vessels in the skin and intestines contract, sending extra blood to the muscles, where it is wanted (that is why people turn 'pale with fright').

Healthy adrenals are responsible for the maintenance of the sodium/potassium balance in the body and, as lack of potassium has been postulated as one major cause of cancer, it is essential to keep this balance correct.

In cases of shock or prolonged stress, adrenaline is produced by the adrenal glands to counter the stress. But byproducts of this adrenaline can result in the formation of free radicals, active carcinogens. Normally adrenaline is balanced with stamina and is a necessary hormone for flight or fight. If one has too much of it in response to non-aggressive situations or emergencies, it is secreted, cannot perhaps be used and it has to be stored in the body. Excessive adrenaline is then a major toxic culprit in all degenerative diseases.

THE PARATHYROIDS

The parathyroids are four small glands at the side of, behind and embedded in the thyroid. These are responsible for maintaining the calcium/phosphorus balance, and in particular in regulating blood calcium. If this falls, then there is muscular spasm of the hands and face; if it rises there may be muscular weakness and diarrhoea. Calcium is then removed from the bones, accumulates in the blood and is excreted, leaving deformed and weakened bones.

THE PINEAL

The pineal gland, near the third ventricle of the brain, is not yet really understood but may be associated with the development of the testes and ovaries. It also seems to be a kind of 'sensory' gland which enables a person to 'orientate' and to sense danger in a different way from the adrenals. The pineal will first sense danger and then pass a message on to the adrenals for action. It has been found in children that those who could orientate well had functioning pineals, while those that couldn't find their way had atrophied pineals. Even at a very early age the pineal gland can atrophy; it can however develop.

THE PANCREAS

The pancreas has the dual role of producing enzymes which go directly into the duodenum, and of producing hormones (in that part of the gland called the islets of Langerhans). Insulin is produced to regulate the blood sugar level, while glucagon increases the production of sugars and turns them into a usable form for the muscles.

Defects in the pancreas will lead to either hypoglycaemia or diabetes.

THE GONADS

The testes and ovaries produce reproductive cells and sex hormones – androgens for males and oestrogens in females – which cause the development of particular male or female characteristics.

THE THYMUS

Science thought for years that the thymus wasted after puberty and had no purpose after that age. Through post-mortems it was noted that the thymus totally calcified after puberty and therefore it was assumed it could not act as a gland; it was found that the thymus was entirely covered by a thick membrane of mucus, surrounded by hardened, fibrous and very tough tissue. It was thought that the master glands regulating all body processes in the body were the pituitary and thyroid glands.

Now science has discovered that the thymus is really an important controller of life. It is known that our immunity depends exclusively on the production of the hormone thymoxin, produced by the thymus, which controls our protective T-helper cells (T cells are so named because they have been produced in the thymus). The body cannot produce T cells if the thymus is not working. These T-helper cells (or lymphocytes) get stored in the bone marrow and when the body faces a crisis of any kind they are released from the bone marrow back into the blood system.

T-helper cells are needed as part of the body's immune response to sudden trauma, accidents, cuts, etc., and, if the thymus is not producing sufficient, disease can set in as the protective elements are not there. If a child, or an adult develops infection, and particularly if it has recurrent infections, it is because the thymus is not producing T-cells and cannot therefore fight infections. It has been shown that there is an 87 per cent survival rate in premature babies who have been strapped to their mothers, thymus to thymus. The thymus gland needs zinc and vitamin A to form lymphocytes (T cells) to fight cancer. A zinc deficiency causes a wasting away of the thymus gland.

It is difficult to stimulate the thymus, but certain soft sounds, like that of the sea, reawaken the capacity of the thymus gland to produce lymphocytes. The thymus also responds to warmth and to percussion. An extraordinarily easy way of stimulating the thymus is to lightly bang the chest rapidly and rhythmically, while thinking about the particular organ that needs help, reinforced by uttering deep Oooos, Mmmmmms, Rrrrrrs. The homoeopathic remedy Viscum album also has a reputation for stimulating the thymus and lymphocyte production.

It is estimated that 96 per cent of the population in fact have a deficient thymus. Even babies are born with a deficient thymus due to genetic weaknesses.

THE THYROID

The thyroid is an endocrine gland located in front of the neck just below the Adam's apple (thyroid cartilage); it has one lobe on each side of the trachea, connected by a bridge (isthmus). The thyroid manufactures two hormones, T_4 thyroxine, which is slow acting, and T_3 thyroxine, which is formed from T_4. An essential ingredient of these hormones is iodine, extracted from the bloodstream.

Thyroid hormones regulate the metabolic activity of the body cells and tissues and influence how the body uses food by regulating the metabolism of sugar, protein and fat, i.e. too little of the hormones means body cells work at too slow a rate. The thyroid gland's actions are regulated by the pituitary gland's thyroid-stimulating hormone (TSH or thyrotrophin), which in turn is regulated by the hypothalamus gland TRH (thyrotrophin-releasing-hormone), which depends on feedback levels of T_3 and T_4 in the bloodstream.

There are a number of thyroid diseases. Hyperthyroidism (or thyrotoxicosis) is when there is an excessive amount of the two thyroid hormones present in the bloodstream. Graves disease is the main cause, i.e. there is an increased secretion of hormones from a gland that is being overstimulated by thyroid-stimulating antibodies, causing the thyroid to enlarge. There are many symptoms:

- Tiredness, extreme nervousness, irritability.
- Palpitations and onset of atrial fibrillations, with increased heart rate, perhaps up to 200 (tachycardia).
- Increased sweating, increased in hot weather; warm moist skin.
- Pruritis (itching skin).
- Loose bowels.
- Voracious appetite, but still loses weight (possible remedy to consider would be homoeopathic iodum).
- Protrusion of eyeballs (exophthalmus), which denotes overactivity of the gland, i.e. 'starey' eyes, patient has a startled or frightened look.
- Throbbing carotids; headaches; unable to relax.
- Muscular tremors, particularly after exertion; check outstretched fingers for tremors.
- Sleeplessness; digestive disorders, diarrhoea.
- Uterine derangements.
- Diminished sugar tolerance; makes diabetes much more severe.
- Metabolic rate increased.
- Often runs in families; mainly in females (10:1) aged 15 to 30, men 30 to 45.

- Symptoms are decreased by administration of thyroxin (pure iodine), which is necessary for proper metabolism of fats and is required to stop the deposition of fat on arterial walls (atherosclerosis or hardening of the arteries).
- There is too much iodine in the blood.
- Toxic nodular goitre (toxic adenoma) develops in people with previous goitre.

Non-toxic goitre (enlargement of thyroid gland) means the gland is not manufacturing excess thyroid hormones T_4 and T_3. It is caused by iodine deficiency, and may be associated with other autoimmune diseases such as pernicious anaemia. Simple goitre (idiopathic goitre) has an unknown cause; the treatment is to use iodised salt (potassium iodide or Lugol's solution or kelp may provide too much iodine). Note that a goitre rarely disappears when only iodine is given, as iodine has no effect on scar tissue; it is necessary to give vitamin E as well.

Hypothyroidism (underactivity of the thyroid gland) is usually caused by Hashimoto's autoimmune thyroiditis; this is the most common cause in areas that are not deficient in iodine. This is when lymphocytes come to regard thyroid tissues as 'foreign', attack, and gradually destroy it by about the age of 58. Alternatively, it is due to inadequate secretion of thyroid hormones, with inefficient production of thyroxin, a lack of iodine and possibly as a result of fluoride intake which decomposes iodine. It may be caused by drugs, spinal luxations, pressure on nerves by contracted muscles, and is sometimes associated with defective kidneys. In thyroid deficiency the level of cholesterol increases in the bloodstream. It is formed in about 15 women, but only one man, in every 1,000. Symptoms include:

- Physical and emotional tiredness; unsmiling face.
- Frequent yawning.
- Dry skin; coarse skin; cold skin; pallor of skin and lips.
- Weakness, lethargy, slow speech and movement; vertigo.
- Decreased sweating; sensation of cold.
- Oedema of eyelids, face and feet.
- Constipation; loss of appetite.
- Impaired short term memory; nervousness; depression, slowing of mental activity.
- Laboured or difficult breathing; breathless even when sitting.
- Heart enlargement; slow pulse.
- Angina, and intermittent claudication.
- High cholesterol level, giving narrowing of arteries (atheroma).
- Brittle nails; burning or tingling sensations.

- Muscle weakness and pain; pains in legs, from the ankle up to the knee.
- Mild persistent aches and pains of unknown cause.
- Excessive menstruation.
- Deafness; hoarseness; loss of hair; gain in weight.
- Pain in chest under sternum, under both ribs, in axillae.
- Backache in lumbar area and between scapula.
- Note if there is any family history of pernicious anaemia or if patient has had vitiligo.

There is a temperature test for hypothyroidism:

- Immediately on waking in the morning place a thermometer in the armpit for 10 minutes.
- If the temperature is below 97.8°F it indicates the possibility of low thyroid activity.
- With women the first test should be made on the second and third days of menstruation.
- In children, two minutes of rectal temperature is adequate; oral temperatures are often misleading as any respiratory infection, sinusitis, etc., will elevate the mouth temperature while the rest of the body may be normal.

Hypothyroidism slows the healing process anywhere in the body, as digestion, assimilation and elimination are slowed down, reducing the speed with which toxins are carried away. Due account should be taken of this when assessing progress of any ailment. Temporary or constant inactivity of the thyroid gland may result in chronic headaches, through nerve and brain poisoning. Deficient activity also leads to accumulation of nitrogenous waste in the system, leading to respiratory troubles such as asthma.

Cancer of the thyroid may result from undue exposure to X-rays of the head, neck and chest, or treatment by X-rays of birthmarks on the face or neck. It may produce asymmetrical lumps on the thyroid, which are hard, round, nodular, and often painless; these will metastasise to other parts of the body and only when, perhaps, a bone breaks for no apparent reason will cancer be suspected. Alternatively the gland may enlarge, be tender, with red inflammatory skin round it.

Over- or under-activity of the thyroid may make it difficult to conceive. During pregnancy and at menopause it is common for the thyroid to enlarge a little – use sea salt, etc., to control it.

Myxoedema is a defect in the thyroid gland, a defect in nutrition. The symptoms include:

- Shrunken thyroid gland; swollen subcutaneous and connective tissues throughout the body.
- Chronic migraine headaches.
- High susceptibility to diseases in general.
- More common in women between 30 and 50 (6:1).
- If there is any irregularity in menstrual flow, check for hypothyroidism.
- Frequent infections.
- Face swollen, features coarse; expression dull and unrelieved by any passing emotions or interests.
- Skin generally dry and yellow, but cheeks are usually bright red in contrast.
- Skin may be swollen, and pit on pressure.
- Skin disorders, e.g. psoriasis, eczema, boils.
- Water retention.
- Hair brittle, thin and harsh.
- Hands become 'spade-like'; feet also large.
- Gait ungainly, slow and deliberate.
- Constipated.
- Always feel chilly; subnormal temperature; cold hands and feet.
- Lowered systolic blood pressure.
- Pulse slow and regular, 50–60 per minute.
- Profound depression.
- May lose a third of the eyebrows.

There are many homoeopathic treatments for thyroid disorders, including the following:

- Hyperthyroidism – pilocarpus, lycopus, iodum CM (4 only), nat. mur., thyroidinum, belladonna, spongia, bromium, fucus tincture, strophantus, kali iod., calc. carb., merc. lycopodeum, nat. ars. if there is a feeling as if thyroid were compressed between thumb and finger, nat. carb. with hard swelling of thyroid.
- Hypothyroidism – kali carb.; also supplementation with iodine and/or L-tyrosine, both of which are necessary in the body's production of thyroxine.
- Cretinism – thyroidinum.

Thyroid diseases use up calcium, so supplements may be required due to lack of iodine which controls calcium balance in the body.

THE LIVER

The liver is the largest organ in the body. There are two lobes, the right one being six times the size of the left one. It is situated at the top of the abdomen on the right side mainly, fitting just under the concave surface of the diaphragm.

Digested food passes through the intestinal wall and goes via the portal veins to the liver for further processing. Of the blood arriving at the liver, 80 per cent comes via the portal veins from the stomach, intestines, pancreas and spleen, and 20 per cent from the hepatic arteries. Once the blood has passed through the liver it leaves via the hepatic veins to the inferior vena cava, and back to the heart.

The liver's main purposes are as follows.

- It produces bile, to emulsify fats and fat-soluble vitamins. This is a continuous process, the bile going via the hepatic duct into the duodenum. If digestion is not going on, any surplus bile is stored and concentrated (up to ten times) in the gallbladder, which is attached underneath the right lobe of the liver. Bile also helps the absorption of food in the intestines, and destroys poisonous organisms, such as micrococci, to prevent excessive decomposition and smell. Most of the bile is reabsorbed with the food nutrients into the bloodstream and returns, via the blood system, to the liver.
- It produces certain proteins required by the blood plasma.
- It converts ammonia, from the used-up tissues of the body, into urea by combining it with carbon dioxide (CO_2), for excretion via the kidneys.
- It produces heat to keep the body temperature constant.
- It produces vitamin B12, to prevent anaemia.
- It produces the anticoagulant heparin, and fibrinogen.
- It stores glucose in the form of glycogen. This can be reconverted to glucose and then passed into the bloodstream when required, to preserve body heat and muscle power.
- It stores fats, which are changed to forms more readily broken down eventually into water and CO_2, or combined with proteins and used as an energy source.
- It stores large quantities of blood.
- It stores vitamins A, B, B12, D, E, K and haemoglobin.
- It detoxifies the blood and renders certain drugs and bacterial poisons (toxins) harmless.

- It extracts iron from the breakdown products of haemoglobin.
- It uses amino acids, some of which are turned into carbohydrates to give readily available energy.

The digestive process generally liquefies solid foods and breaks them down to simpler substances, i.e. proteins become amino acids which the liver re-arranges so that they are assembled into proteins that the human body can use. If, however, an essential amino acid is missing then proteins cannot be efficiently made – only complete proteins can be used to build or repair tissues. Fats become fatty acids and glycerol, starches become simple sugars, both of which are then available as fuel to give the body energy. Waste products can be converted into useful substances, or changed so that they can be excreted so as to prevent any accumulation in the tissues.

Malfunction of the liver may result in:

- Nausea, digestive disturbances, flatulence; lack of energy, mental lethargy, insomnia and malnutrition.
- High blood pressure.
- Haemorrhages, ulcers, piles, etc.
- The skin becomes jaundiced.
- The liver becomes hard and painful to touch.

Any delay in getting rid of waste products can result in almost any ailment.

In cancer patients, a chronically damaged liver is common; the liver then fails to purify the blood or to reactivate oxidising enzymes. Both of these functions can be helped by the proper diet.

The liver is adversely affected by artificial chemicals in food. A diet free of animal proteins is perhaps the most important factor in the regeneration of a damaged liver. The bile system is greatly stimulated by caffeine absorbed into the liver via the colon (i.e. through coffee enemas).

PIIMA YOGHOURT

Piima yoghourt was developed in Finland and arrived in the UK in 1987. It consists of a number of powerful organisms, including *Lactobacillus acidophilus* and *L. bulgaricus, Streptococcus thermophilus, bifidobacteria,* and *amophilus.* It therefore covers a very wide spectrum of beneficial bacteria similar to those in the intestines and, like the intestines, piima predigests any proteins eaten and carries the 'building blocks', i.e. amino acids, into the bloodstream to be made into human protein. It is therefore helpful, whenever eating protein, to have some Piima yoghourt beforehand to break these proteins down. It has a very gentle action and can quickly affect the internal bacteria. It has a high level of acidophilus, so there is no need to take any supplementary acidophilus as well.

The intestinal flora, consisting as it does of over 300 different species and weighing between 3 and 4 lb, have innumerable functions to perform and are crucial to the body's immune system and its detoxification. The beneficial bifidobacteria need to be kept up to strength to counter the tendency of putrefactive bacteroides bacteria to increase; certain factors, such as the use of antibiotics, either taken directly or indirectly through meat and dairy products, tend to favour the increase of bacteroides. Major stresses may also upset the balance between the various types of bacteria.

The putrefactive bacteria have, of course, a part to play; the job of the bacteroides, the coliforms, salmonella and *E. coli* is to rot or disintegrate matter in the intestines, at the same time producing foul gases. Diets high in animal protein favour these bacteria, which will increase at the expense of the desirable *bifidobacteria* and *Lactobacillus bulgaricus, L. acidophilus* and *Streptococcus thermophilus.* Constipation favours bacteroides proliferation.

Insufficient digestion in the stomach leading to undigested protein molecules entering the small intestine encourages the overgrowth of the yeast/fungus candida, with its resultant toxic metabolites passing through the intestinal wall into the lymph and bloodstream. It is therefore essential to do everything to encourage the growth of the beneficial bifidobacteria, particularly after any course of antibiotics.

Piima is very effective at breaking down the tough lining of glutenous substances formed in the small intestine as a result of candida infestation, but it may have to be taken regularly for many months before it has any significant impact. Piima, which is a protein food in itself, should be taken on its own or at least half an hour before a meal, to act as a bedding for the food and to allow it time to get into the gut before the food arrives. As it is a protein it can be taken, under the Hay system of combining foods, with other proteins such as nuts. Virtually any amount may be taken. It is not necessary to have the yoghourt on its own all the time.

PROCEDURE FOR MAKING PIIMA YOGHOURT

- Decide on a culturing area where the temperature will stay between 72°F and 75°F. This is most important. If it gets above 80°F it will separate into curds and whey, and if it goes below 69°F it will become stringy and slimy. However, even then not all is lost and it only needs to be kept for some hours more and it will tend to thicken up. When put into the fridge it will thicken up even more. It is useful to have a maximum/minimum thermometer to monitor the temperature of the area in which the Piima is being grown. With a little experimentation and imagination one can organise an area, box, airing cupboard, etc., which will fulfil these conditions. The heat from an electric light bulb in a box can be sufficient.
- Do not heat or use a yoghourt maker as this will kill the Piima.
- Use glass containers rather than plastic.
- Keep jars and lids very clean; sterilise them in boiling water first.
- Use freshest, preferably whole, unpasteurised cows' milk (although, when experienced, one can use goats' milk, which will be slightly thinner), or canned, evaporated or even dried milk.
- Avoid contamination by airborne bacteria (probably the most common cause of failure to produce perfect Piima every time) or from aerosols, household fumes, insecticides, pest strips, sprays, paint fumes, dusts, moulds, yeasts, tobacco smoke, etc.
- When starting with powder starter (which may not be available in the UK but which should have been stored in the refrigerator on receipt), pour one cup of fresh milk into the jar and add the contents on the foil package. Put the lid on the jar, shake until it is mixed and place in culturing area.
- When starting with already mixed yoghourt, take one tablespoon and mix it well into a pint of milk and place in culturing area. It is as simple as that.
- Check 24 hours later to see if it is coagulated; if not, leave for up to another 12 hours. When coagulated place in fridge at once, where it will thicken up a bit more.

The Piima is now ready to eat, and also to use as a starter for further supplies. It is prudent at this stage to take a tablespoonful of the fresh yoghourt as a starter for further supplies and follow the above procedure. This ensures that you have not contaminated the fresh yoghourt through opening it up several times, and also ensures that you know you have a fresh supply before the first lot is finished. Piima can remain stable in a refrigerator for weeks.

Piima can be made from goats' milk, although it is more difficult to get it thick. If you buy goats' milk frozen, defreeze it quickly by putting the bag in a container with some hot water and then make the yoghourt, which should then come out thicker.

Suggestions for ways of using Piima yoghourt are:

- First thing in the morning, half an hour before any breakfast.
- Before any protein meal.
- With seeds, nuts, avocados, with yolk of egg, with vegetable bouillon.
- As a dip with celery.

Do not take it with either grains or fruit, because of their sugar content.

CAPRICIN

Capricin is an anti-fungal fatty acid derived from caprylic acid in coconuts. It was developed by an American biochemist, Dr Tobin Neesby, for the effective treatment of the fungal yeast *Candida albicans*. By encasing the caprylic acid in a substance that can pass undamaged through the acid in the stomach (enteric coating), the capsule releases its contents slowly in the place where it is most needed, i.e. the intestines, particularly the small intestine, where most of the candida yeast thrives. Here it kills the majority of the candida organisms but does not harm the friendly bacteria. Capricin Forte, as supplied by BioCare, also supplies highly bioavailable calcium and magnesium. It is perfectly safe to use, unlike nystatin, which is liable to have certain side effects.

Initial doses of Capricin will kill off many candida fungi, causing a die-off effect as extra toxins (mainly aldehydes) are released by the dead candida in the gut. This may result, during the first few days, in flu-like symptoms, bloated stomach, headaches, fatigue, etc. It is therefore better to start with a low dose and increase when there is no adverse reaction.

The recommended dosage is:

- First week, one capsule (400 mg) three times a day before meals.
- Second week, two capsules three times a day before meals.
- Third week, three capsules three times a day before meals until carton is finished.

A fat of some sort, such as milk, butter, salad oils, etc., should be included in each meal when Capricin is taken, and it should be taken with plenty of liquid.

This programme may have to be repeated once or twice, depending on each individual's response. Once it produces diarrhoea or very loose stools for some long period then it can be assumed that it is working satisfactorily.

Acidophilus (500 mg) or Vitalplex should be taken routinely after the first week of Capricin treatment to start repopulating the gut with friendly bacteria. Better still take Piima yoghourt before each meal as this has four other friendly bacteria as well in strong concentrations.

As antibiotics are a potent cause of candida proliferation, Capricin can be taken as a prophylactic (one a day) during long-term antibiotic treatment, together with *L. acidophilus* (or a combination of bacteria as in

Piima yoghourt) to repopulate the intestinal flora that the antibiotics have been responsible for getting rid of.

USEFUL ADDRESSES

For further information or supplies, contact BioCare Ltd, 20-24 High Street, Solihull, West Midlands B91 3TB, tel. 021-705 4975.

DIFLUCAN

Diflucan is a fluconazole antifungal agent manufactured by Pfizer Laboratories. Clinical trials appear to indicate greater efficacy than that of other antifungal drugs.

When colonies are systematically invasive, fungi are very difficult to eradicate. Diflucan is now routinely used in the management of the immunocompromised patient, especially while undergoing treatment after surgery and when catheter feeding takes place.

Details and further information can be obtained from Pfizer Laboratories.

CHIROPHONETICS

Chirophonetics is a form of gentle massage on the back with essential oils, combined with certain specific sounds aimed at reaching deeply into a person's innermost spiritual levels. It is based on ideas of Rudolf Steiner, as outlined in his philosophy called anthroposophy, and the theory is too involved to outline here. Nevertheless, the proof of the pudding is in the eating and some remarkable benefits have been felt by people who have been treated by this system, regularly used by patients at Springhill.

Basically it is felt that communication between individuals can only happen through the medium of speech. There are, of course, various body movements and eye contacts that have meaning between individuals, but to communicate properly requires some kind of language, some sound.

The sounds used in chirophonetics are adjusted according to the personality of the patient, as shown initially by their outlook and character. But their responses are also noted to various massage movements and sounds which indicate, to a trained chirophonetician, the weaknesses or strengths of the patient and whether they can operate in the astral sphere (similar to the state one is in when almost asleep), when the body responds readily to commands consciously given it – in fact whether they can work in a higher spiritual sphere. For instance the sound of MMMMMMMM is a soothing sound, linking the spirit with the body. The sound OOOOOOO is connected with the bone structure, and therefore is used more when treating, say, handicapped children. The sound RRRRRRRR connects the physical with the astral body. These vibrations of sound reach deep into the body lymph system, into the circulation. It has been found very successful with children with asthma.

Like many other natural medicine methods of treatment, chirophonetics aims at balancing the body's energies, although here it is balancing spiritual, rather than the purely physical energies that are balanced in, say, acupuncture. The object is to harmonise the four bodies (or energies) of the earthly, the etheric, the astral and the I or ego. Once in harmony, things begin to change in the body. Many people feel stronger inwardly. Some find relief from pain. Some find they have an impulse to do things differently and have overcome something lacking in their lives up to that point.

If one can think of one's objectives, then feel it inwardly, and lastly go and practise it, then the three functions will act together for success. Unfortunately chirophonetics is not a technique one can practise on oneself, although mothers have soon been taught the basic method for treating their children for specific ailments. Being individuals we have, ourselves, to consciously contact our ego or I, get away from the purely physical side of life and use and get the benefit of the power of our spiritual natures.

HOMOEOPATHY

Homoeopathy is based on the principle that 'like cures like'. Where a poisonous substance can produce certain symptoms when administered to a healthy person, it will, when homoeopathically prepared (potentised) and diluted, cure an illness which produces similar symptoms. Homoeopathic remedies are completely safe in the dilutions normally given, are non-addictive and free from deleterious side effects. They are not suppressive in any way but rely entirely on stimulating a person's own defensive mechanisms, and helping the body to heal itself.

Cancer is a whole body constitutional ailment and, as such, requires constitutional remedies. These are remedies which are matched to the personality of the patient more than the physical symptoms he may have and are usually prescribed at the start of any treatment. As this is a big subject, fully covered in the homoeopathic literature, I suggest readers who are interested should refer to a book like *The Principles and Art of Cure by Homoeopathy* by Herbert A. Roberts.

Having said that, there are a number of remedies which have a specific bearing on various organs, and many of them have been found to be beneficial against various types of cancers. In 1893 a very well-known successful homoeopath, J. Compton Burnett, wrote a book entitled *Curability of Tumours by Medicines*, which detailed cases of cancers cured through the use of homoeopathic remedies. As these remedies are as effective now as they were then, anyone with cancer should consider the possibility of long-term cure through the use of these remedies.

The following list is given merely to direct your attention to possibly helpful remedies, which can then be followed up by referring to a *Homoeopathic Materia Medica* such as the excellent and easily understood one by Boericke. Only some of the outstanding characteristics of each remedy are given as a guide to the most relevant remedy, and the help of a qualified experienced homoeopath should be sought.

- Acetic acid (3–30 C) for epithelial cancers. The epithelium is the cellular layer covering the skin and inner surface of hollow organs such as bowels, bladder, stomach, intestines, and of the secreting glands and air passages.
- Adrenaline (1M), one dose to help the detoxification process when there is any hyperactivity of the adrenals which would produce excess cortisone. Such excess holds up excretion of sodium, which then builds up and becomes toxic.

- Alumen, for epithelioma, scirrhus of the tongue – hardening of tissues of tongue, ulcers with indurated base.
- Argentum metallicum for cartilage thickening and infiltration. For scirrhus cancer (a hard form of cancer in which much fibrous tissue develops, e.g. in the breast or uterus). For ulceration of the stomach with radiating pains.
- Arsenicum album is for cancer of the stomach and/or uterus; for epithelioma of the lip, face and tongue. Sharp burning pains are very typical of anyone for whom this remedy will help, as are exhaustion and weakness. It is useful after an operation, to stop a recurrence of the cancer. There is always restlessness and everything is worse at night. The patient is fastidious.
- Asterias rubens is for cancer of the breast with acute and lancinating pains. The axillary glands are swollen, hard and knotted; there are hard painful lumps in the breast. It is particularly for flabby, red-faced people with lymphatic constitutions. The symptoms are worse at night, and in damp weather.
- Aurum met. is for cancer of the nose and lip; for people with suicidal tendencies and for those who are depressed.
- Aurum mur. is for cancer of the tongue which is hard as leather.
- Aurum mur. natronatum (3x) – one of the best remedies for uterine cancers. High blood pressure is often found in people for whom this remedy is suitable.
- Bellis, where tumours have resulted from bruises, blows or falls. It helps where there is any form of mechanical pressure, e.g. enlarged hearts, pregnancies and uterine fibroids.
- Berberis is useful for kidney, bladder and liver problems, particularly if there are wandering pains.
- Bismuth is for cancer of the stomach, when there are burning pains, hard lumps between the navel and the edge of the lower ribs on the right side, and the patient vomits all fluids.
- Bromium is for tumours in the breast with stitching pains; they are worse on the left side and for pressure.
- Bufo is for cancer of the uterus, breasts and ovaries, although it is probably only palliative. It sometimes suits the feeble-minded, prematurely senile, or epileptic.
- Cadmium sul. is for cancer of stomach. It helps persistent vomiting, and burning and cutting pains, and is recommended for the general health of cancer sufferers.
- Calcarea acetica is for cancer pains.
- Calcarea oxal. is for excruciating pains of open cancers.
- Caltha palustris tincture is for uterine cancer.

- Carbo animalis (30 C) is for cancer of the uterus, with burning pains down the thighs, and of the forehead; there will be symptoms of great weakness and want of energy, prostration, glandular swellings in the axillary, inguinal and mammary regions, and a putrid taste and discharges. For excessive bloating use 200 C.
- Cadmium sul. is for carcinoma of the stomach. It helps the persistent vomiting, and the burning and cutting pain in the stomach.
- Carcinosin is for cancer of the uterus and mammary glands, with great pain and induration. It is particularly indicated where there is a family history of cancer, in which case it should be used in conjunction with other remedies. It is recommended for fastidious personalities (cf arsenicum album), and is indicated where there has been a severe reaction to vaccinations.
- Calc. ars. is for cancer of the pancreas – it helps relieve pain. It is also recommended for cancer of the uterus, with burning pains, and for epileptics.
- Ceanothus is a spleen remedy when there is pain generally on the left side, and for anaemic patients.
- Chelidonium majus is a liver remedy where there is an outstanding symptom of pain under the inferior angle of the right scapula, or alternation of diarrhoea with constipation.
- Chimaphila umbellata is for cancer of the breast, with atrophy, in women with very large breasts, particularly if there are sharp pains.
- China (*Cinchona officinalis*) is particularly indicated where there has been a loss of vital fluids through bleeding or diarrhoea. The liver and spleen may be swollen.
- Cholesterinum is for cancer of the liver (1M upwards).
- Cicuta virosa, 3x six-hourly, where a tumour is not very sensitive to pressure, or where there is great pain in the arm with rigidity and loss of power.
- Cistus canadensis is for cancers of the glands of the neck and of the breasts, if there is a cold feeling everywhere, or if there is glandular fever.
- Clematis erecta is for cancer of the breast, where there are swollen glands and where the patient is very sensitive to the cold.
- Condurango is for stomach cancers and epithelioma of the lips or anus. It detoxifies sodium carbonate excess. A noteworthy sign that this may be the right remedy is the appearance of painful cracks in the corners of the mouth. There may be a stricture in the oesophagus, where food seems to stick. It allays the pain of gastralgia accompanying cancer of the stomach.

- Conium is for cancerous diathesis (general liability to cancer), for cancer of the glands, lips, face, stomach, breasts (especially if, at every menstrual period, the breasts become large, sore and painful), uterus, bones, if there is great weakness, heartburn or spasms of the stomach. It is indicated for ill effects of shock to the spine that are worse from any jar or walking, for muscular weakness, or burning, stinging pains, and for complaints due to blows or contusions (cf bellis).
- Crotalus horridus is for cancer of the stomach with vomiting, for cancer of the tongue and uterus. It is indicated if the patient haemorrhages easily, and if the disease is markedly worse on the right side.
- Euphorbium relieves the burning pains of cancer for 5–6 hours, particularly pains in limbs and paralytic weakness in joints. It is used for ulcerating carcinoma and epithelioma of the skin.
- Fuligo ligni is for cancers of the tongue, scrotum, womb and for epithelial cancers.
- Galium aparine tincture is for cancerous ulcers and hard tumours of the tongue. It is said to have the power of suspending or modifying cancerous action.
- Graphites is for gastric ulcers, cancers of the stomach and the intestines.
- Hekla lava is for bony cancers.
- Hydrastis is for cancers where pain is the principal symptom: for cancer of the stomach, where the patient vomits everything except water mixed with milk; for cancer of the rectum, with constipation and haemorrhoids; for catarrh anywhere; for epithelioma of the skin; for cancer of the breast; and particularly for people with a jaded look, sallow complexion, loss of appetite, chronic constipation.
- Iodum is for cancer of the uterus, when the patient only feels well when eating but, despite this, progressively loses weight.
- Kali arsenicum is for skin cancers with malignancy without external signs, where there are numerous small nodules under the skin.
- Kali cyanatum (200 C) is for cancer of tongue and ulcers; it is particularly for the patient who cannot masticate on account of agonising neuralgia.
- Kreosote is for cancer of the uterus, with burning in the pelvis; it is also for breast cancer that is hard, bluish-red and covered with scurvy protuberances.
- Lachesis (CM) is for cancers of the breast, ovaries, uterus, stomach, when they are bluish or purplish with great pain; the patient wakes

up feeling worse, may faint if constricted, or in a warm bath, and is markedly worse on the left side.

- Lapis albus is for the pre-ulcerative stage of carcinomas of the skin, for cancer of the uterus with haemorrhages, and for fibroid tumours.
- Lycopodeum is for epithelioma of the lip and for carcinomas in general.
- Mercurius is for profuse odorous perspiration and breath; painful, slimy and bloody stools; and for ulcerations of the mouth and nose.
- Mezereum is for cancer of the stomach, where there is great emaciation (often the result of suppression of eruptions); the patient is very sensitive to cold air, and suffers from violent retching and vomiting.
- Muriaticum acidum is for cancer of the tongue; the tongue is leathery with hard lumps, and the patient may suffer from haemorrhoids.
- Natrum muriaticum is for when there is great weakness that is worse in the morning; for blinding headaches and a cold body; the symptoms get worse from heat.
- Phosphorus is for cancer of the womb and the breast; the patient may also suffer from pancreatic diseases or a congested liver, and feel better for cold.
- Phytolacca tincture is for cancer of the breast; the breast is hard, painful and purple. It is also for cancer of the lips. It is pre-eminently a glandular remedy, for many throat problems, quinsy, tonsillitis, for shooting pains, like electric shocks, and for people with a tendency to fatness, sluggish circulation, lazy disposition.
- Psorinum – Burnett often used this psora constitutional remedy at the start of treatment, often followed by thuja, as he knew most patients had been vaccinated at one time or another.
- Radium is for epithelioma, when there is itching all over the body, a burning of skin as if from a fire, and when there is necrosis and ulceration of the skin.
- Rumex acetosa is for epithelioma of face, and for cancer of the bowels and oesophagus.
- Ruta is for carcinoma of the lower bowel, when there is prolapsus ani every time the bowels move.
- Sanguinaria is for cancer of the rectum.
- Scirrhinum is a cancer nosode for general cancerous diathesis (a predisposition to cancer); for enlarged glands; and for cancer of the breast.
- Sempervivum tectorum is for cancer of the tongue, with ulcers,

when there is bleeding easily; it is also for mammary carcinoma.

- Sepia is for cancer of the rectum, when there is an upward tendency of symptoms – all pains are from below up.
- Tarentula cubensis is for the atrocious pains of cancer, for the pains of death; it is said to soothe the last struggle. It is also used when there is a purplish hue, and for cancer of the breast.
- Thuja is for when tumours have come as a result of vaccinations.
- Viscum album (low) is to prevent cancer cell proliferation and metastasis; it restores normal enzyme and hormone metabolism through stimulating the thymus and lymphocyte production. It also relieves the pain of tumour growths, and, as a tincture is used in Iscador.
- X-ray is for cancer of the skin in people exposed to X-rays, and for leukaemia.

BACH FLOWER REMEDIES

Dr Edward Bach was a Welshman, born in 1886, whose whole life was dedicated to finding a system of healing which would use natural means – he was convinced, from a very early age, that there must be such a system. He had an overwhelming compassion for any person, bird or animal in trouble and decided he wanted to be a doctor. After a frustrating three-year period in his father's factory, he joined the Worcestershire Yeomanry where he could indulge his love of the open air and of nature study. He was still desperately wanting to be a doctor and eventually his father agreed he should go to Birmingham University, going on to University College Hospital in London and qualifying in 1912.

He hated London life but was a workaholic, working day and night. He soon came to realise that the best way of seeing how disease worked was to study, not his books, but the patients, and he noticed that:

- Some patients reacted well to a certain remedy, some to another.
- Patients with a similar personality or temperament would often respond to the same remedy, while people with different personalities responded best to other remedies.

This made him realise that the personality of the patient was of more importance than the bodily symptoms in his treatment. At this time he had not heard of homoeopathy, in which Hahnemann was also convinced that 'mentals' were more important in guiding one to the correct remedy than the physical manifestations of a disease. In his study of patients he saw much suffering in the process of healing and he felt certain that true healing should be gentle and painless.

Bach progressed and started practising in Harley Street, making a lot of money, but he was still dissatisfied with the current orthodox methods of treatment, and joined University College Hospital as an assistant bacteriologist in order to look for the answer to his problems. There he found that intestinal germs which were normally in the gut increased significantly when a person had a disease, producing intestinal toxaemia. (This is in line with current thinking about the effect of candida in excessive quantity in the gut in all degenerative diseases.) He then made a vaccine from these bacilli which was injected into patients

– who recovered from their chronic illnesses. These vaccines were widely used by orthodox medical men. This was satisfactory, but Bach believed that it should be unnecessary to have to inject these vaccines.

Bach accordingly started preparing oral vaccines from the bacilli in the gut. These were called the Bach nosodes (and were prepared in the homoeopathic manner). He named seven groups of bacilli:

- Proteus.
- Dysentery.
- Morgan.
- *Faecalis alkaligenes.*
- *Coli mutabile.*
- Gaertner.
- No 7.

These 'vaccines' cleansed the intestinal tract, resulting in a general improvement in the patient's health. These nosodes were in themselves remarkable discoveries and, even if Bach had not progressed further, his discovery of these nosodes was enough to demonstrate his genius.

While considering these nosodes, Bach was at the same time noting the 'mentals' of the patients. He realised that definite types of personalities belonged to each group and these seven groups corresponded to seven different types of personality. Being able to prescribe according to the personal traits of the patient was far less harassing than working from physical examinations, and Bach worked extremely hard to classify the symptoms to be found under these seven groups according to the personalities of the patients. These 'vaccines' or nosodes improved a patient's general condition to such an extent that their particular ailments disappeared.

Bach realised that his seven nosodes only covered ailments under Hahnemann's miasm of psora, and that there were other chronic diseases that had to be treated. He also did not really like using disease products, and believed there must be some purer method of treatment – somewhere in nature there was the answer. He did in fact find that the vibrations of the plant the star of Bethlehem (*Ornithogalum umbellatum*) were similar to those of chronic ailments treatable by the Morgan nosode.

At this time he became gravely ill (probably with cancer), became unconscious, was operated on while he was unconscious, and was subsequently given three months to live. However, he continued with his work more furiously than before in order to finish it before the end of his three months, but found himself getting better. He decided that it was his absorbing purpose in life, which did not give him time to think about his own ailments, that had helped him regain his health.

In 1919 he was given the post of bacteriologist at the London Homoeopathic Hospital, where he read Hahnemann's *Organon*. He then realised that he and Hahnemann were working along the same lines, as Hahnemann had, some 100 years earlier, discovered that:

- Each case of illness required individual treatment according to the individuality of the patient.
- One should treat the patient, not the disease.
- One should use the temperament of the patient as a guide to the remedy required, quite irrespective of the physical complaint.
- Remedies were more beneficial when they were only repeated after any improvement from an earlier dose had ceased.
- Hahnemann had concluded that one, or a combination, of three poisons had to be eliminated before a complete cure of a chronic complaint could be achieved. These were his 'miasms' – syphilis, sycosis (or gonorrhoea) and psora. Bach came to the conclusion that his intestinal toxaemia was identical to Hahnemann's psora.

Bach realised that everyone belonged to one of a number of fairly obvious group 'types', where each member had roughly the same kind of personality and temperament which were recognisable by their behaviour or moods or attitude, and he wondered if everyone in one group would have the same sort of diseases. He then came to the intuitive realisation that everyone belonging to a particular type would not have the same diseases, but would react to a particular ailment in more or less the same way.

He realised that disease is due primarily to certain disturbed states of mind which lead to disturbed bodily functions, as of course the mind is in complete and automatic charge of the mental and physical conditions of a person. Any continued worry, therefore, would cause some disorganisation in the physical body. Bach stressed the importance of being happy, by which he meant the individual should be living life to the full, guided by instinct and intuition; the person should have a certain spontaneity and be uninfluenced by others, and thereby able to be of the greatest help and service to his fellow men. Bach himself was entirely guided by his intuition.

The knowledge that a state of mind was responsible for the physical illness would do much to dispel fear of disease. Moods, of course, change, thus requiring a change of remedy. He also realised that the signs of an approaching disease were clearly shown beforehand by the person's particular state of mind, and treatment could be given even before signs of the illness were apparent.

Bach proposed that an inharmonious state of mind is the primary cause of sickness. He considered that defects such as pride, cruelty, hate, self-love, ignorance, instability, greed, all had repercussions on the physical condition of a person. For example:

- Pride is arrogance and rigidity of mind, and this will give rise to those diseases which produce rigidity and stiffness in the body (arthritis).
- Cruelty results in pain.
- Hate results in loneliness, temper, mental nerve storms and hysteria.
- Ignorance and a persistence in refusing to see the truth leads to shortsightedness and impairment of vision and hearing.
- An unstable mind will lead to unstable movement and coordination.
- Greed leads to diseases of the stomach.
- Frustration over unfulfilled ambitions may lead to thrombosis.

It is therefore necessary to trace back any ailment to the possible mental causes that started it. Without getting neurotic, it is useful to notice changes that are indications that something is wrong – when one should pause and consider, in order to prevent further complications.

During his search for the later remedies Bach suffered from various states of mind that he wanted to find a remedy for, and many of these states of mind were accompanied by great physical sufferings. This required great courage and dedication and left Bach physically weak. Among Bach's sayings that arose at this time are the following:

- Disease is but the consolidation of a mental attitude.
- It is certain that a personality without conflict is immune from illness.
- Boredom is responsible for much more disease than would be generally realised.
- Fear of disease is really self-interest, for when we are earnestly absorbed in the welfare of others there is no time to be apprehensive of personal maladies.
- There is no true healing unless there is a change in outlook, peace of mind, and inner happiness.
- Take no notice of the disease – think only of the outlook on life of the one in distress.
- Long-continued fear or worry depletes vitality and the body loses its natural resistance to disease.

Similarly, in conventional homoeopathy it has been found that the mental symptoms of a patient are more important to consider and cure than the particular manifestation of the illness such as fever, palpitations, pain, etc., which will be cured once the 'mentals' have been treated. No notice is taken of the nature of the disease. The individual is treated and he becomes well – then the disease goes. It is a familiar phenomenon in homoeopathy that when a patient says he is feeling better – even though his symptoms are the same – then he is on the way to recovery.

Dr Bach looked for remedies that would restore vitality to the sick and enable them to overcome their mental worries, fears or depressions and assist in their own healing. It is the patient, not the disease, which needs treatment. Indeed, he went further and considered that disease can be prevented before its actual physical symptoms appear, by overcoming any negative states of mind.

Remedies need changing as moods or states of mind change. There may be apparent worsening of physical symptoms or a change of symptoms, but the correct remedy to give at that time is the one that most nearly corresponds to the mood of the patient and his outlook. For example, a person who has been lacking confidence (for which larch is the remedy) may gain confidence, possibly too fast, and he may take on too much too quickly, becoming exhausted and depressed – a different state of mind, requiring a different remedy (perhaps mustard).

The body has a natural in-born resistance to disease, but this appears to be weakened through negative states of mind. The remedy lies within ourselves. Negative thoughts actually poison the system – they hinder the effectiveness of any treatment.

THE DEVELOPMENT OF THE REMEDIES

Bach flower remedies are homoeopathic remedies, but with a difference. These remedies are not really 'like curing like'. They would not, like all other homoeopathic remedies, cause any symptoms if taken in a gross form. But they are similar in that they can produce the feeling of the mental symptoms in a sensitive person, and thereby can be used to cure those symptoms in anyone. They are a simple and natural method of healing through an individual's personality. Bach was 'led' by his extreme sensitivity and intuition – as if he were dowsing – to use flowers, for no scientific reason.

Bach was very sensitive and so acute did his quality of sensitivity become that when he placed the petal of a flower on his tongue the emotional and mental imbalances that the bloom could cure manifested themselves in his own being. In this way he was able to classify the feelings each flower produced, thus enabling him to pick out the flowers that produced each of these feelings in himself. So were born the Bach flower remedies. He would only take the finest flower-heads, i.e. that part that held the potential seed, and he found the sun's heat was essential in the process of extracting the healing power. He laid these flower heads in a saucer of water and found the water was impregnated with the healing 'essence'.

Bach had the power to heal through touch. Indeed, he was so sensitive that he could tell what disease his next patient was suffering from, even before they arrived. This was a very personal power, but he wanted others to have this power too, and if this was impossible he wanted to give them some simple remedies which would have similar powers of healing.

He started off with three flowers – impatiens, mimulus and the wild clematis – and he started treating people with these three remedies whenever he found they fitted the personality types he divined these flowers would cure. Thus, impatiens was used for the impatient person, with extreme mental and therefore muscular tension; mimulus for people with fears of things like illness, pain, accidents etc.; while clematis was for the dreamy, sleepy, impractical, absent-minded person.

In 1930 Bach gave up all his paying practice in order to search for other flowers that would cover the other groupings of people that he had been observing and classifying closely. He was often poor, but was spurred on by his all-consuming desire to find a system of medicine which would be simple, pain-free and effective.

Dr Bach first discovered 12 states of mind (marked with an asterisk, *, in the following list), to which he added other helper remedies, making in all 38 separate negative states of mind under seven groupings:

- Fear.
- Uncertainty.
- Insufficient interest in present circumstances.
- Loneliness.
- Oversensitivity to influences and ideas.
- Despondency or despair.
- Over-care for welfare of others. (This last heading seems more positive than negative and could I think be better called self-love or self-concern.)

These subdivisions appear to cover most of the major behavioural patterns that can be called negative states of mind.

FEAR

- No 26, rock rose* – an extreme state of fear; almost paralysing fear; real, temporary terror; panic; extreme fright. Suitable for people who have been fearful all their lives.
- No 20, mimulus* – normal kind of fear of everyday worldly things of a known origin, such as going to the dentist, illness, pain, accidents, poverty, darkness, of being alone, of misfortune, of death. Claustrophobia. Shy; blush easily; afraid of people; ill at ease in a crowd (agoraphobic).
- No 6, cherry plum – fear of mental weaknesses, of going round the bend, of doing fearful things, of reason giving way, of harming others or ourselves; fear of suicide. A feeling of desperation in certain situations.
- No 2, aspen – groundless fear of vague unknown unexplainable terrors. Feeling of agitation, perhaps on waking out of sleep. Fears unrelated to anything. To shake with fear. Can be with a person all the time. Often for children with nightmares.
- No 25, red chestnut – fears and anxiety for other people, perhaps for one's children when out, for family if anything happens to one, for people on the TV, for someone who is very ill.

FOR THOSE WHO SUFFER UNCERTAINTY

- No 5, cerato* – for those lacking confidence in themselves; self-distrust; those who are weak, who follow the advice of others, e.g. trying out various medicines; talkative; asking questions about what to do but not listening to the answers. For those who doubt their own ability or wisdom, who think everyone else knows best. Wistful, would like to be like others. Very intuitive people. Mistrust their own judgment.
- No 28, scleranthus* – for those unable to take decisions, who cannot make up their minds, who suffer extremes of energy/apathy or optimism/pessimism; who get travel sick. Hesitant and uncertain. For those who are 'standing still' and don't know why things are not happening. For those who are quiet. Symptoms keep changing. Moody; 'grasshopper minds'.
- No 12, gentian* – for those easily discouraged, doubtful and disheartened with a negative outlook. Give up easily at any setback. Will pick themselves up for a time, but will receive another setback and become depressed again. Lack of faith in life, pessimistic. Worry about everything and have a negative attitude to everything.

Look for trouble. Depressed from known causes.

- No 13, gorse – for those who feel completely hopeless and in despair of ever getting better. Useful where a person has given up hope, e.g. in last stages of cancer. More extreme than gentian. Fear of death. Usually has sallow complexion with dark rings round eyes.

- No 17, hornbeam – for those uncertain of their ability to cope; who are tired in mind mainly, but also in body (Monday morning feeling); a disinclination to do anything unless it is of supreme interest (cf olive, which has extreme tiredness and would not have the strength to do anything). A bit lazy – do not want to get on with the job. A supporting or helper remedy.

- No 36, wild oat – for those uncertain of what to do in life, doubtful of how to fulfil their vague ambitions. Weak, despondent types, though talented: dissatisfied. A remedy for anyone who feels they have not achieved their goal in life, who is frustrated because they are not doing what they want to do, e.g. they may be unemployed, although they will try many things. Very unhappy and depressed. Frustration may lead to congestion, e.g. thrombosis.

INSUFFICIENT INTEREST IN THE PRESENT

- No 9, clematis* – daydreamers, drifters, absent-minded, no interest in life; poor memories, sleepy, impractical, indifferent; a child who dreams at school; artistic people who create mentally; feelings of unreality. For those who look forward to death. Useful in cases of fainting or unconsciousness, when it can be rubbed into gums, behind ears, on wrists and palms.

- No 16, honeysuckle – for those who live in the past, nostalgic; have regrets for things they should have done or not done; homesick; pessimists about the future. Very useful for bringing people into the present.

- No 37, wild rose – those who become resigned to their fate and unwilling to make any effort; perhaps have been told there is nothing more to be done and they accept the verdict. Apathetic; not a feeling of hopelessness, just acceptance of the position; always weary; dull company.

- No 23, olive – those who have suffered much mentally and physically and cannot make any further effort. Completely exhausted; daily life is an effort (even shaving), and without pleasure. Restores vitality in convalescence. A great pick-me-up, this is a great strengthener, e.g. helpful after flu, childbirth, etc.

- No 35, white chestnut – those whose persistent unwanted worry-thoughts stop them from enjoying the present and interfere with their peace of mind, i.e. the gramophone-record minds. Brings peace of mind, e.g. after emotional rows that keep on turning over and over in the mind, occupying the mind to the exclusion of everything else.
- No 21, mustard – those who are moody, perhaps with black depression, like a cloud that descends, remains and then lifts; or despair without apparent reason. Cf Gentian if it is depression from known reasons; sweet chestnut if it is anguish and depression from the heart; cherry plum if the depression is suicidal. Egocentric; melancholic.
- No 7, chestnut bud – those who do not benefit from experience and tend to make the same mistake over and over again; always rushing; failure to learn by experience. Remedy for ailments that happen at the same time every year, i.e. the same beliefs come up time and time again, so the same illnesses come up – 'calendar beliefs'.

LONELINESS, SELF-CENTREDNESS

- No 34, water violet* – those who prefer to be alone, enjoy their own company, keep themselves to themselves; capable and self-reliant; great tolerance of others; quiet, serene, calm, talented; aloof; not usually afraid of anything. Often feel superior to others, but they do not interfere with them, only think they are superior. Pride may manifest itself as physical stiffness and tension, but not all stiffness means this remedy will help.
- No 18, impatiens* – those who are impatient with others and therefore prefer to work alone; prefer independence; extreme mental tension like a vice on their head; also some muscular tension; quick mentally and physically; know where they are going; accident-prone; like to overtake on the road; upset nervous digestion; irritable, quick flashes of temper.
- No 14, heather – those who cannot bear to be alone for long and are always seeking companionship; 'buttonholers'; love to talk about their complaints. Tiring to the listener. Egocentric; full of self-concern.

OVERSENSITIVE TO OUTSIDE INFLUENCES AND IDEAS

- No 1, agrimony* – sensitive, happy, ebullient, peace-loving people, optimists, who are distressed by arguments or quarrels and do all they can (even to taking alcohol or drugs to excess) to bear their trials with cheerfulness. Appear not to have a care in the world. Worry concealed from others, being hidden behind an outward cheerfulness. Strong in themselves, but may appear weak through giving in for the sake of peace. Like company; the life and soul of the party. Restless; insomnia; mental or physical torture. A remedy for pain, and to bring peace to the body or mind.

- No 4, centaury* – the servile type, weak-willed and weak in body; 'doormat' types; sweet, gentle people, over-anxious to serve others. Always thinking about others. Never complain. Timid, docile; too easily influenced by others. Attract bullies or more powerful characters through their subservience. A very negative state.

- No 33, walnut – those with definite ideals but who may be tempted away from their life ambitions or way of life by opinions of even stronger personalities; oversensitive to ideas. For those undergoing big changes in their lives, such as puberty, menopause, new jobs, schools, marriage, etc.

- No 15, holly – those who are attacked by, and suffer from, thoughts of jealousy, envy, suspicion, revenge, vexation. An antidote for hatred; for feelings of discontent that everyone experiences from time to time; for desire for revenge. Active intense types. Angry and resentful children. Counteracts feelings of selfishness.

FOR DESPONDENCY OR DESPAIR

- No 19, larch – those who expect to be failures and do not consider they are as good or capable as others. No self-confidence, despite considerable ability; feel inferior to others. Useful before an exam or driving test, etc., i.e. against fear of failing, despondency.

- No 24, pine – those who blame themselves, whether warranted or not; self-reproach, guilt complex; over-conscientious; a feeling of unworthiness; givers rather than receivers. Never satisfied; lack of love for themselves.

- No 11, elm – efficient, hold positions of trust or any responsibility; indispensable. Occasionally think they cannot complete their task in life, and they therefore feel weak, exhausted, and temporarily inadequate.

- No 30, sweet chestnut – extreme mental anguish, heartbreak, hopelessness and terrible despair, e.g. bereavement; at end of their tether for some reason, but would not consider suicide (like cherry plum which has a more unstable kind of despair) as they are people of strong character, who keep their distress to themselves and do not talk about their problems (similar to agrimony).

- No 29, star of Bethlehem – those who are in great despair as a result of conditions which, for a time, bring great unhappiness, sadness and grief. After-effects of shock or grief, whether immediate or long-term, mental or physical (possibly unrealised shock).
- No 38, willow – those who feel they don't deserve, and resent, their bad fortune (cf holly, which is more outgoing, willow being more introverted) and become embittered with failure. 'Wet blankets', depressed; self-centred. Take without giving. Feeling of 'things not being fair'; sulky; 'dog in the manger' (cf chicory).
- No 22, oak – for those continually struggling against great odds and ill health, who are despondent and discontented with themselves if illness interferes with their lives; ceaseless in their efforts to find a cure when they are sick; do not like being ill; never lose hope; get despondent but feel somewhere there must be an answer. The opposite of gentian, which gives up easily. Patient; persistent; reliable, dependable people who like to help others, but are not doormats. Full of commonsense.
- No 10, crab apple – for those who feel despair and disgust; who feel mentally and physically unclean through some trivial or more serious disease, e.g. something like eczema; who feel despondent if treatment fails. Over-conscientious on trivial matters; fussy. To cleanse the system of toxins accumulated during shock, hatred or anger. Children who have been born with eczema may be helped with this remedy (and possibly star of Bethlehem for any possible shock or trauma).

OVER-CARE FOR WELFARE OF OTHERS

This encompasses self-love and self-concern, as well as self-denial.

- No 8, chicory* – self-love, self-pity, desire for attention; those over-possessive of others and have a need to influence others; use emotional blackmail to achieve their ends. Worrying over trifles, fretful.
- No 31, vervain* – those with strict principles who are convinced they must convert all around them. Like to work with others (unlike impatiens, who wish to work on their own). Fanatics, reformers. Strong characters, organisers; lots of natural energy; full of ideas. Highly strung; perhaps unable to sleep; stress, strain, physical tension, over-work through over-enthusiasm; perfectionists; workaholics.

- No 32, vine – those who are very capable, ambitious and feel it their duty to direct and dominate others. Inflexible, crave power. Bullies, but underneath may crumble if challenged; domineering; want everything done their way. Dogmatic; single-minded; inflexible. Ambitious, quick thinkers.
- No 3, beech – intolerant people who tend only to look for others' faults and criticise them. Generally lack humility; never see good in anyone; always fault-finding; arrogant, think they know everything (cf chicory). Therefore lonely. Intolerant of physical conditions, e.g. wind, cold, etc.
- No 27, rock water – those who are very strict in their way of living, with strong opinions and high ideals; fanatical; deny themselves many of the joys and pleasures of life as they consider it would interfere with their life, i.e. self-repression, self-denial, self-martyrdom. Very up-tight people.

RESCUE REMEDY

This is ideal for the following:

- For use in emergencies, such as after an accident or at the onset of a sudden illness during a journey.
- For shock, physical or mental.
- To calm a person before a traumatic experience, e.g. pre-exam nerves, before taking off on a flight.
- To prevent panic and have a calming influence, such as at the start of whooping cough.
- To ease the pain and depression of a terminal illness.

Rescue remedy is a composite of five remedies, all aimed at the results of shock. It is made up of:

- Star of Bethlehem (no 29), for shock.
- Rock rose (no 26), for terror and panic.
- Impatiens (no 18), for mental stress and tension.
- Cherry plum (no 6), for desperation.
- Clematis (no 9), for the bemused, faraway feeling.

The Rescue Remedy can also be applied externally, after dilution, to burns, bruises, cuts, sprains, pains. And for pain relief Rescue Remedy is available as an ointment.

However, if the patient looks as if he is not responding to treatment, or looks as if he needs a number of remedies, give either holly (no 15) to active intense types or wild oat (36) to weak despondent types.

HOW TO USE BACH FLOWER REMEDIES

Mix two drops of stock solution from up to five chosen remedies in a water (90 per cent)/alcohol (10 per cent) mixture. Then give four drops in a teaspoon of water or milk direct on the tongue four times a day for best results. Hold in the mouth for a moment before swallowing. Or give two drops in half a glass of water or fruit juice and sip fairly frequently over a period of a few hours. Remedies can be used on children or animals in exactly the same way according to their nature, and can also be used on plants.

Remedies will work very quickly on temporary moods, within an hour or two, but it may take longer to counteract a negative state of mind that has persisted for a long time, depending on the person. The healing process starts immediately and it is often people close to us who see a change before we are aware of one ourselves.

USEFUL INFORMATION

For further information contact the Dr Edward Bach Centre, Mount Vernon, Sotwell, Wallingford, Oxon. OX10 0PZ. Also see page 272.

CASE HISTORY TAKING

It is always helpful for any practitioner if a new patient comes prepared with the answers to questions about his or her medical background. When faced with questions about what happened in the past, many people suffer a mental blackout, but if these questions are thought about quietly at home beforehand there is more chance of the answers becoming available. Patients going to Springhill are asked to supply the following information, and it would be useful for any potential patient anywhere to have the answers to these points in mind before seeing their doctor or other medical practitioner.

Firstly, they are asked for factual information covering date of birth, occupation, marital status, any family, next of kin, name of general practitioner and specialist, if any.

Then as much information about their present complaint; when it started, does anything make it better or worse, how is it progressing. The pattern of the progress of the illness is often very illuminating and helps the medical staff to gauge what stage the illness has reached.

Then information about past illnesses and operations chronologically, including major ailments of near family. This will suggest any hereditary weaknesses that will have to be taken into account.

What drugs or treatment are they, or have they been, subject to, including, in particular, antibiotics? This may also be illuminating, as repeated courses of antibiotics may have increased candida infestation. What vitamin/mineral/herbal supplements have they been taking, if any?

Then questions about lifestyle – diet itemised over a day, cigarettes smoked, alcohol, amount of sugar, tea and coffee taken, cravings and allergies, known or suspected.

Physical details of symptoms of pain, coughs, bowel and urinary complaints, female problems, nervous system weaknesses, etc. Weight and height, and whether there have been obvious changes in weight.

Patients are also asked to summarise their most significant life events and traumas, present stresses, future hopes. This is a reflection of the importance of the mind over the body, and how stresses can vitally affect the functioning of the body. This is very much in accord with the homoeopathic view, that mental symptoms are more important than the purely physical ones in finding a cause and, hopefully, a cure for the disease. Almost anything is relevant when trying to assess the reasons behind a chronic disease, so patients should be prepared for what some people consider an unusual experience. To a homoeopath in particular, the most insignificant and, on the surface, irrelevant details of any peculiar symptoms are of the greatest value.

FURTHER
READING

An End to Cancer, Leon Chaitow (Thorsons, 1978)

Cancer/Leukaemia and Other Seemingly Incurable Diseases and *Advice for the Prevention and Treatment of Numerous Diseases, Including Cancer and Leukaemia*, Rudolf Breuss (W. Margeiter, 1982)

Fresh Hope in Cancer, Maurice Finkel (Health Science Press, 1978)

A Gentle Way With Cancer, Leon Chaitow (Thorsons, 1978)

A Time to Heal, Beata Bishop (Severn publishers, 1985)

'How Killer Cells Kill', *Scientific American*, January 1988, 258.1

'Inside Science', *New Scientist*, March 24, 1988

Nutrition
The Bristol Diet, Dr Alec Forbes (Century, 1984)

The Complete Sprouting Book, Per and Gita Sellmann (Turnstone Press, 1981)

Add a Few Sprouts, Martha H. Oliver (Keats Publishing, 1975)

Gluten Intolerance, Good Health Guide (Keats Publishing, 1987)

The Miracle Nutrient Coenzyme Q10, Dr Emile G. Bliznakov and Gerald L. Hunt (Thorsons, 1988)

Superoxides and Their Effects, Dr Yukie Niwa (H.B. Johnson Woodier Ltd.)

Good Food, Gluten Free, Hilda Cherry Hills (Roberts Publications, 1976)

Food Combining For Health, Doris Grant and Jean Joice (Thorsons, 1984)

Fit for Life, Harvey and Marilyn Diamond (Bantam, 1985)

Cancer Prevention Diet, Michio Kushi (Thorsons, 1984)

Cancer and Its Nutritional Therapies, Dr Richard A. Passwater (Keats Publishing, 1978)

Felmore Ltd Health Publications, Numbers 82, 97, 98, 111, 133

Bach Flower Remedies
The following books are all published by C.W. Daniel Co. Ltd:

The Medical Discoveries of Edward Bach, Physician, Nora Weeks, 1973

Handbook of the Bach Flower Remedies, Philip M. Chancellor, 1971

The Twelve Healers and Other Remedies, Edward Bach, 1933

Heal Thyself, Edward Bach, 1931

Bach Remedies Repertory, F.J. Wheeler, 1952

Introduction to the Benefits of the Bach Flower Remedies, Jane Evans, 1974

Homoeopathy
Homoeopathy Materia Medica, William Boericke (Boericke & Runyon, 1927)

Homoeopathic Insight into Cancer, Causes, Treatment and Cure, Dr S.A.M. Bihari (B. Jain Publishers, 1982)

The Principles and Art of Cure by Homoeopathy, Herbert A. Roberts (Health Science Press, 1936)

Tumours of the Breast: Treatment and Cure and *Curability of Tumours by Medicine*, J. Compton Burnett (B. Jain publishers, 1893)

Awareness Through Movement, Moshe Feldenkrais (Penguin, 1972)

Protection For Life, Dr Yukie Niwa and Maurice Hanssen (Thorsons, 1989)

Bring Out the Magic in Your Mind, Al Koran (Tandem, 1964)

Guide to Self Healing, Matthew Manning (Thorsons), 1989

Practice of Autosuggestion by the Methods of Emile Coue, C. Harry Brooks (OUP); *Self-Mastery through Conscious Autosuggestion*, Emile Coue (George Allen & Unwin, 1922)

Love, Medicine and Miracles, Bernie S. Siegel (Rider, 1986)

Getting Well Again, Carl Simonton (Bantam, 1978)

The Stress of Life, Hans Selye (McGraw Hill, 1956)

Anatomy of an Illness, Norman Cousins (Penguin, 1979)

Maximum Immunity, Michael A. Weiner (Gateway, 1986)

Free Radicals in Biology and Medicine, Barry Halliwell and John M.C. Gutteridge (Clarendon Press, 1989, 2nd edition)

Radiation and Health, R. Russell Jones and Richard Southwood (Wiley, 1989)

Iron in Immunity, Cancer and Inflammation, Maria de Sousa and Jeremy H. Brock (Wiley, 1989)

Candidiasis, Gerald P. Bodey and Victor Fainstein (Raven Press, 1985)

REFERENCES

Bayer, A.S., Edwards, J.E. and Seidel, J.A., (1976) 'Candida meningitis' *Medicine*, 55: 477–486

Bennett, J.E., (1974) 'Chemotherapy of systemic mycoses' *N. Engl. J. Med.*, 290: 30–32

Bodey, G.P., (1966) 'Fungal infections complicating acute leukaemia' *J. Chron. Dis.*, 19: 667–687

Bodey, G.P., DeJongh, D., Isassi, A. and Friereich, E.J., (1969) 'Hypersplenism due to disseminated candidiasis in a patient with acute leukaemia' *Cancer*, 26: 417–420

Bodey, G.P., and Luna, M., (1974) 'Skin lesions associated with disseminated candidiasis', *J.A.M.A.*, 229: 1466–1468

Bodey, G.P., Rodriguez, V., Chang, H.Y. and Narboni, G. (1978), 'Fever and infection in leukaemic patients. A study of 494 consecutive patients' *Cancer*, 41: 1610–1622

Bodgen, E. and Kessell, J., (1937) 'Monilial meningitis', *Arch. Pathol.*, 223: 909–912

Bondestam, S., Jansson, S.E., Kivisaari, L., Elonen, E., Ruutu, T. and Anttinen, I., (1981) 'Liver and spleen candidiasis: Imaging and verification by fine-needle aspiration biopsy' *Br. Med. J.*, 282: 1514–1515

Braude, A.I. and Rock, J.A., (1959) 'The syndrome of acute disseminated moniliasis in adults' *Arch. Intern. Med.*, 104: 93–100

Brincker, H., (1983) 'Prevention of mycosis in granulocytopenic patients with prophylactic ketoconazole treatment' *Mycosen.* 26: 242–247

Caroline, L., Rosner, F. and Kozinn, P.J., (1969) 'Elevated serum iron, low unbound transferrin and candidiasis in acute leukaemia' *Blood*, 34: 441–451

Carpentieri, U., Haggard, M.E., Lockhart, L.H., Gustavson, L.P., Box, Q.T. and West, E.F., (1978) 'Clinical experience in prevention of candidiasis by nystatin in children with acute lymphocytic leukaemia' *Journal of Pediatrics*, 92: 592–595

Cherubin, C.E., Boden, M., Kavaler, F., Lerner, S. and Cline, W., (1968) 'Infective endocarditis in narcotic addicts' *Annals of Internal Medicine*, 69: 1091–1098

Chesney, P.J., Teets, K.C., Mulcihill, J.J., Salit, I.E. and Marks, M.I., (1976) 'Successful treatment of candida meningitis with amphotericin B and 5-fluorocytosine in combination' *Journal of Pediatrics*, 89: 1017–1019

Chesney, P.J., Justman, R.A. and Bogdanowicz, W.M., (1978) 'Candida meningitis in newborn infants; a review and report of combined amphotericin B-flucytosine therapy' *Johns Hopkins Medical Journal*, 142: 155–160

Chmel, H., Grieco, D.P., Odds, F. and Mitchell, C., (1980) 'Candida osteomyelitis; report of a case' *American Journal of Medical Sciences*, 266: 299–304

Clarke, M., Davies, D.P., Odds, F. and Mitchell, C., (1980) 'Neonatal systemic candidiasis treated with miconazole' *British Medical Journal*, 281: 354

Craddock, V.M., (1987) 'Effect of the trichothecene mycotoxin diacetoxyscirpenol on nitrosamie-induced oesophageal cancer and on relevant enzymes in oesophagus and liver' *IARC-Sci-Publ*, 84: 266–269

Craddock, V.M., Hill, R.J. and Henderson, A.R., (1987) 'Stimulation of DNA replication in rat oesophagus and stomach by the trichothecene mycotoxin diacetoxyscirpenol' *Cancer-Lett*, 38: 199–208

Curry, C.R. and Quie, P.G., (1971) 'Fungal septicaemia in patients receiving parenteral hyperalimentation' *New England Journal of Medicine*, 285: 1221–1225

Dennis, D.L., Peterson, C.G. and Fletcher, W.S., (1968) 'Candida septicaemia in the severely traumatized patient' *Journal of Trauma*, 8: 177–186

Eilard, T., Alestig, K., Beskow, D., Norrby, R. and Whalen, P., (1978) '5-Fluorocytosine-amphotericin B treatment in disseminated mycoses' *Current Chemotherapy: Proceedings of the 10th International Congress of Chemotherapy*, 220–222, American Society for Microbiology, Washington D.C.

Evans, G.W. and Johnson, P.E., (1978) 'Relative zinc availability in human breast milk, infant formulas, and cow's milk' *American Journal of Clinical Nutrition*, 31: 416–421

Felman, Y.M. and Nikitas, J.A., (1979) 'Trichomoniasis, candidiasis and

Corynebacterium vaginale vaginitis' *New York State Journal of Medicine*, 79: 1563–1566

Fishman, L.S., Griffin, J.R., Sapico, F.L. and Hecht, R., (1972) 'Hematogenous candida endophthalmitis, a complication of candidemia' *New England Journal of Medicine*, 286, 675–681

Fudenberg, H.H., (1971) 'Genetically determined immune deficiency as the predisposing cause of "autoimmunity" and lymphoid neoplasia' *American Journal of Medicine*, 51, 295–298

Giombetti, R., Hagstrom, J.W.C., Landey, S., Young, M.C. and New, M.I., (1971) 'Cushing's syndrome in infancy. A case complicated by monilial endocarditis' *American Journal of Diseases of Children*, 122, 264–266

Goldberg, P.K., Tessler, S., Lenoral, R.A.K. and Kozinn, P.J., (1979) 'Incidence and significance of candida in bronchial aspirates' *American Society for Microbiology, Annual Meeting*

Gottlieb, S., Khuddus, S.A., Balooki, H., Dominguez, A.E. and Myerburg, R.J. (1974) 'Echocardiographic diagnosis of aortic valve vegetations in candida endocarditis' *Circulation*, 50: 826–830

Griffin, J.R., Pettit, T.H., Fishman, L.S. and Foos, R.Y., (1973) 'Blood-borne candida endophtalmitis. A clinical and pathologic study of 21 cases' *Archives of Opthalmology*, 89: 450–456

Haris, L.J., (1960) 'Further observations on a simple procedure to eliminate thrush from hospital nurseries' *American Journal of Obstetrics and Gynecology*, 80: 30–31

Hart, P.D., Russell Jr, E. and Remington, J.S., (1969) 'The compromised host and infection. II. Deep fungal infection' *Journal of Infectious Diseases*, 120: 169–191

Haruda, F., Bergman, M.A. and Headings, D., (1980) 'Unrecognized candida brain abscess in infancy. Two cases and a review of the literature' *Johns Hopkins Medical Journal*, 147: 182–185

Hermans, P.E., Ulrich, J.A. and Markowitz, H., (1969) 'Chronic mucocutaneous candidiasis as a surface expression of deep-seated abnormalities' *American Journal of Medicine*, 47: 503–519

Hersh, B.M., Gutterman, J.U., Mavligit, G.M., Mountan, C.W., McBride, C.M., Burgess, M.A., Lurie, P.M., Zelen, M., Takita, H. and Vincent, R.G., (1976) 'Immunocompetence, immunodeficiency and prognosis in cancer' *Annals of the New York Academy of Sciences*, 276: 386–406

Higgs, J.M. and Wells, R.S., (1972) 'Chronic mucocutaneous candidiasis: associated abnormalities of iron metabolism' *British Journal of Dermatology*, 86 (Supplement 8): 88–102

Holder, I.A., Kozinn, P.J. and Law, E.J., (1977) 'Evaluation of candida percipitin and agglutinin tests for the diagnosis of systemic candidiasis in burn patients' *Journal of Clinical Microbiology*, 6: 219–223

Jordan, W.M., Bodey, G.P., Rodriguez, V., Ketchel, S.J. and Henney, J., (1979) 'Miconazole therapy for treatment of fungal infections in cancer patients' *Antimicrobial Agents and Chemotherapy*, 16: 792–797

Klein, J.D., Yamauchi, T. and Horlick, S.P., (1972) 'Neonatal candidiasis, meningitis and arthritis; observations and a review of the literature' *Journal of Pediatrics*, 81: 31–34

Knight, L. and Fletcher, J., (1971) 'Growth of *Candida Albicans* in saliva: stimulation by glucose associated with antibiotics, corticosteroids and diabetes mellitus' *Journal of Infectious Diseases*, 123: 371–377

Kozinn, P.J., Taschdjian, C.L., Dragutsky, D. and Minsky, A. (1962) 'Enteric candidiasis. Diagnosis and clinical considerations' *Pediatrics*, 30: 71–85

Kozinn, P.J., Caroline, L. and Taschdjian, C.L., (1964) 'Conjunctiva contains factor inhibiting growth of *Candida Albicans*' *Science*, 46: 1479–1480

Law, E.J., Kim, O.J., Stieritz, D.D. and MacMillan, B.G., (1972) 'Experience with systemic candidiasis in the burned patient' *Journal of Trauma*, 12: 543–552

Lehner, T., (1964) 'Candidal fungaemia following extraction of teeth and its relationship to systemic candidiasis' *British Dental Journal*, 117: 253–256

Lehrer, R.I., (1971) 'Inhibition by sulfonamides of the candidacidal activity of human neutrophils' *Journal of Clinical Investigation*, 50: 2498–2505

Lipton, S.A., Kickeuy, W.F., Morris, J.H. and Loscalzo, J., (1984) 'Candidal infection in the central nervous system' *American Journal of Medicine*, 76: 101–108

REFERENCES

Littman, M.L., Horowitz, P.L. and Swadey, J.G., (1958) 'Coccidioidomycosis and its treatment with amphotericin B' *American Journal of Medicine*, 24: 568–592

Lopez, E. and Alterman, K. (1968) 'Intra-uterine infection by candida' *American Journal of Diseases of Children*, 115: 663–670

Louria, D.B., Buse, M., Brayton, R.G. and Finkel, G., (1966) 'The pathogenesis of *Candida tropicalis* infections in mice' *Sabouraudia*, 5: 14–25

Louria, D.B., Shannon, D., Johnson, G., Caroline, L., Okas, A. and Taschdjian, C.L., (1967) 'The susceptibility to moniliasis in children with endocrine hypofunction' *Transactions of the Association of American Physicians*, 80: 236–249

Lowder, J.N., Lazarus, H.M. and Herzig, R.H., (1982) 'Bacteremias and fungemias in oncologic patients with central venous catheters. Changing spectrum of infection' *Arch. Intern. Med.*, 142: 1456–1459

Lowenthal, R.M., Grossman, L., Goldman, J.M., Storring, R.A., Buskard, N.A.S., Park, D.S., Murphy, B.C., Spiers, A.S.D. and Galton, D.A.G., (1975) 'Granulocyte transfusions in treatment of infections in patients with acute leukaemia and aplastic anaemia' *Lancet*, 1: 353–358

Maksymiuk, A.W., Thongprasert, S., Hopfer, R., Luna, M., Fainstein, V. and Bodey, G.P., (1984) 'Systemic candidiasis in cancer patients' *American Journal of Medicine*

Marks, M.L., Marks, S. and Brazeau, M., (1975) 'Yeast colonization in hospitalized and non-hospitalized children' *Journal of Pediatrics*

Masur, H., Rosen, P.P. and Armstrong, D., (1977) 'Pulmonary disease caused by *Candida* species' *American Journal of Medicine*, 71: 363–370

Meberg, A., Langslet, A., Sovde, A., and Kolstad, A., (1977) 'Candida septicemia with choriorentinitis, osteomyelitis and arthritis treated with systemic miconazole and intra-articular amphotericin B' *Mykosen*, 20: 257–260

Medoff, G., Comfort, M. and Kobayashi, G.S., (1971) 'Synergistic action of amphotericin B and 5-fluorocytosine against yeastline organisms' *Proceedings of the Society for Experimental Biology and Medicine* 138: 517–574

Merz, W.G., Evans, G.L., Shadomy, S., Anderson, S., Kaufman, L., Kozinn, P.J., Mackenzie, D.W., Protzman, W.P. and Remington, J.S.,

(1977) 'Laboratory evaulation of serological tests for systemic candidiasis: a co-operative study' *Journal of Clinical Microbiology*, 5: 596–603

Meunier-Carpentier, F., Kiehn, T.E. and Armstrong, D., (1981) 'Fungemia in the immunocompromised host' *American Journal of Medicine*, 71: 363–370

Mills, S.A., Seigler, H.F. and Wolfe, W.F., (1975) 'The incidence and management of pulmonary mycosis in renal allograft patients' *Ann. Surgery*, 182: 617–626

Mirsky, H.S. and Cuttner, J., (1972) 'Fungal infection in acute leukaemia' *Cancer*, 2: 348–352

Montgomerie, J.Z. and Edwaards Jr, J.E., (1978) 'Association of infection due to *Candida Albicans* with intravenous hyperalimentation' *Journal of Infectious Diseases*, 137: 197–201

Moynahan, E.J., (1975) 'Zinc deficiency and cellular immune deficiency in acrodermatitis enteropathica in man and zinc deficiency with thymic hypoplasia in Fresian calves: a possible genetic link' *Lancet*, II: 710

Nash, G., Foley, F.D., Goodwin Jr, M.N., Bruck, H.M., Greenwald, K.A. and Pruitt Jr, B.A., (1971) 'Fungal burn wound infection' *J.A.M.A.*, 215: 1664–1666

Nezelof, C., Jammet, M.L., Lortholary, P., Labrune, B. and Lamy, M., (1964) 'L'hypoplasie héréditaire due thymus' *Archives Francaise de Pediatrie*, 21: 897–920

O'Connell, C.J., Cherry, A.C. and Zoll, J.G. (1973) 'Osteomyelitis in cervical spine. *Candida guilliermondii*' *Annals of Internal Medicine*, 79: 748

Parker Jr, J.C., (1980) 'The potentially lethal problem of cardiac candidosis' *American Journal of Clinical Pathology* 65: 991–1000

Parker Jr, J.C., McCloskey, J.J. and Knauer, K.A., (1976) 'Human cerebral candidiasis. A postmortem evaluation of 19 patients' *Human Pathology*, 12: 23–28

Parker Jr, J.C., McCloskey, J.J. and Knauer, K.A., (1976) 'Pathobiologic features of human candidiasis. A common deep mycosis of the brain, heart and kidney in the altered host' *American Journal of Clinical Pathology*, 65: 991–1000

Pillay, V.K.G., Wilson, D.M., Ing, T.S. and Kark, R.M., (1968) 'Fungus infection in steroid-treated systemic lupus erythematosus' *J.A.M.A.*, 205: 261–265

Pockros, P.H. and Silberman, H., (1962) 'Parenteral nutrition complicated by candidiasis' *Journal of Infectious Diseases*, 145: 592–593

Ray, T.L., (1987) 'Oral candidiasis' *Dermatol-Clin.*, 5(4): 651–662

Rifkind, D., Marchioro, T.L., Schneck, S.A. and Hill Jr, R.B., (1967) 'Systemic fungal infections complicating renal transplantation and immunosuppressive therapy. Clinical, microbiologic, neurologic and pathologic features' *American Journal of Medicine*, 43: 28–38

Rose, H.D., (1978) 'Venous catheter-associated candidemia' *American Journal of Medicine*, 275: 265–269

Rosenbaum, R.B., Barber, J.V. and Stevens, D.A., (1974) '*Candida albicans* pneumonia' *American Review of Respiratory Diseases*, 109: 373–378

Rubin, A. and Alroy, G.G., (1977) '*Candida albicans* abscess of lung' *Thorax* 32: 373–376

Salter, W. and Zinnerman, H.H., (1976) 'Bacteremia and candida septicaemia' *Minnesota Med.*, 50: 1489–1499

Sams Jr, W.M., Jorizzo, J.L., Snyderman, R., Jegasothy, B.V., Ward, F.E., Weiner, M., Wilson, J.G., Yount, W.J. and Dillard, S.B., (1979) 'Chronic mucocutaneous candidiasis. Immunologic studies of three generations of a single family' *American Journal of Medicine*, 67: 948–959

Sandford, G.R., Merz, W.G., Wingard, J.R. Charache, P. and Saral, R., (1980) 'The value of fungal surveillance cultures as predictors of systemic fungal infections' *Journal of Infectious Diseases*, 142: 503–509

Schacter, J., (1978) 'Chlamydial infections' *New England Journal of Medicine*, 298: 540–548

Schimpff, S.C., Young, V.M., Greene, W.H., Vermeulen, G.D., Moody, M.R. and Wiernik, P.H., (1972) 'Origin of infection in acute nonlymphocytic leukaemia. Significance of hospital acquisition of potential pathogens' *Ann. Intern. Med.*, 77: 707–714

Schonebeck, J., (1972) 'Studies of candida infection of the urinary tract and on the antimycotic drug 5-fluorocytosine' *Scandinavian Journal of Urology and Nephrology Supplement*, 11: 1–48

Seelig, M.S., (1966) 'The role of antibiotics in the pathogenesis of candida infections' *American Journal of Medicine*, 40: 887–917

Seelig, M.S., (1980) 'Magnesium deficiency in the pathogenesis of disease' in *Early Roots of Cardiovascular Skeletal and Renal Abnormalities*, Plenum Medical, New York

Seelig, M.S., (1981) 'Nutritional roots of combined system disorders' in *Clinical Disorders in Pediatric Nutrition*, Marcel Dekker, New York

Shumacher, H.R., Ginns, D.A. and Warren, W.J., (1964) 'Fungus infection complicating leukaemia' *American Journal of Medical Science*, 247: 313–323

Sickles, E.A., Young, V.M., Greene, W.H. and Wiernik, P.H., (1973) 'Pneumonia in acute leukaemia' *Ann. Intern. Med.*, 79: 528–534

Siegel, M., Murphy, M., Counts, G.W. and Meyers, J.D., (1982) 'Prophylactic ketoconazole for the prevention of fungal infection in bone marrow transplant patients' Abstract 166 in *Program and Abstracts 22nd Interscience Conference on Antimicrobial Agents and Chemotherapy*, Miami, October 1982, p.94, American Society of Microbiology, Washington D.C.

Simpson, M.B., Merz, W.A., Kurlinski, J.P. and Solomon, M.H., (1977) 'Opportunistic mycotic osteomyelitis. Bone infections due to *Aspergillus* and *Candida* species' *Medicine*, 56: 475–482

Singer, C., Kaplan, M.H. and Armstrong, D., (1977) 'Bacteremia and fungemia complicating neoplastic disease' *Am. J. Med.*, 62: 731–742

Sjoberg, K.H., (1966) 'Moniliasis – an internal disease? Three cases of idiopathic hypoparathyroidism with moniliasis, steatorrhea, primary amenorrhea and pernicious anaemia' *Acta Medica Scandinavica*, 179: 157–166

Stone, H.H., (1974) 'Studies in the pathogenisis, diagnosis and treatment of Candida sepsis in children' *Journal of Pediatric Surgery*, 9: 127–133

Triger, D.R., Slater, D.N., Goepel, J.R. and Underwood, J.C.E., (1981) 'Systemic candidiasis complicating acute hepatic failure in patients treated with cimetidine' *Lancet*, 2: 837–838

Twomey, J.J., (1973) 'Infections complicating multiple myeloma and chronic lymphocytic leukaemia' *Arch. Intern. Med.*, 132: 562–565

Weinstein, M.P., Reller, L.B., Murphy, J.R. and Lichtenstein, K.A., (1983) 'The clinical significance of positive blood culture. A comprehensive analysis of 500 episodes of bacteremia and fungemia in adults. Laboratory and epidemiologic observations' *Rev. Infect. Dis.* 5: 35–70

Williams, D.M., Krick, J.A. and Remington, J.S., (1976) 'Pulmonary infection in the comopromised host. Part 1' *Am. Rev. Respiratory Diseases,* 114: 359–394

Wingard, J.R., Merz, W.G. and Saral, R. (1979) '*Candida tropicalis*: A major pathogen in immunocompromised patients' *Ann. Intern. Med.,* 91: 539–543

Winston, D.W., Gale, R.P., Meyer, D.V., Young, L.S. and UCLA Bone Marrow Transplant Team, (1979) 'Infectious complications of human bone marrow transplantation' *J. Clin. Invest.,* 58: 1–31

Winter Jr, W.D. and Foley, G.E. (1956) 'Candida infections in children with neoplastic disease' *Pediatrics,* 18: 595–603

INDEX

CANDIDA ALBICANS: YEAST AND YOUR HEALTH
Gill Jacobs

What is Candida albicans?
How is it linked to ME, digestive disorders, cystitis, depression,
menstrual problems, multiple sclerosis?
What can be done to help?

Candida Albicans presents a probing and objective account of how health
problems may develop when the balance of the candida yeast fungus
inside all our bodies is disturbed – often by extensive use of antibiotics,
steroids or the pill, by an unhealthy diet and stress, or by inherited
problems with immunity. On the basis of extensive interviews, Gill
Jacobs evaluates the attitudes and experiences of patients, some of
whom were ill for many years before gaining recognition, as well as
examining the varied approaches to treatment.

ISBN 0 356 18685 7   £5.99 (UK)

ENCYCLOPAEDIA OF NATURAL MEDICINE
Michael Murray and Joseph Pizzorno

The *Encyclopaedia of Natural Medicine* is the most comprehensive guide and reference to the use of natural measures in the maintenance of good health and the prevention and treatment of disease. It explains the principles of natural medicine and outlines their application through the safe and effective use of herbs, vitamins, minerals, diet and nutritional supplements, and covers an extensive range of health conditions, from asthma to depression, from psoriasis to candidiasis, from diabetes to the common cold.

Drawing on the centuries-old wisdom of the healing powers of nature, and supported with modern scientific investigation, the *Encyclopaedia* is the ultimate guide to a natural, healthy lifestyle.

Michael Murray is a leading researcher in the field of natural medicine and a member of the faculty of Bastyr College, one of the world's foremost naturopathic colleges. Joseph Pizzorno is a prominent educator in natural medicine, and the President and co-founder of Bastyr College.

ISBN 0 356 17218 X   £12.99 (UK)

YOUR CANCER, YOUR LIFE
Dr Trish Reynolds

What is cancer?
What are the symptoms?
How can cancer be treated?
What do chemotherapy, surgery, radiotherapy, hormone treatment
involve?
Do certain treatments cause side effects?
What does having cancer mean?

Taking a sympathetic but positive approach, Dr Trish Reynolds, a
cancer specialist with 10 years' experience, provides the comprehensive
information needed by every cancer patient. She explains the different
forms and symptoms of cancer, and examines treatments such as
surgery, radiotherapy and chemotherapy, balancing their benefits
against possible side effects.

With this knowledge, Dr Reynolds encourages you to have the
confidence to make positive choices and participate in managing your
treatment. Rather than handing over control to the 'experts', she
emphasises that *you* are the best judge of what's right for *you*: it's your
cancer and your life.

ISBN 0 356 15417 3   £6.95 (UK)

THE COMPLETE GUIDE TO STRESS MANAGEMENT
Dr Chandra Patel

What is stress?
What are the causes and effects of stress?
Can stress be managed?

Stress is a fact of everyday life. It stimulates activity and creativity, and adds excitement and spice to our lives. But too much stress can have serious implications for our physical, mental and spiritual health and well-being.

In *The Complete Guide to Stress Management*, expert Dr Chandra Patel identifies the causes of stress and how different people respond to them, and examines how stress contributes to the development and exacerbation of numerous illnesses, such as heart disease and high blood pressure. She then provides simple but effective relaxation techniques which counteract and alleviate the harmful effects of stress, and enhance the quality of our lives.

Extensively researched and fully comprehensive, this book is an essential aid to coping with the pressures of modern living.

ISBN 0356 15641 9   £8.99 (UK)

CHOICES IN HEALTH CARE
Elaine Farrell

Whether you need to find a local G.P. or a private specialist, facilities for a home birth or hi-tech maternity care, negotiate the waiting lists or take out health insurance, evaluate long-term or respite care for a relative, this book will guide you around the choices.

Elaine Farrell, a freelance researcher and writer with an NHS background, assesses all the options available to people who want the best possible treatment for themselves and their families. Such guidance will become increasingly important as the changing role of the health services places greater emphasis on customer choice.

Extensively researched, up-to-date and comprehensive, *Choices in Health Care* provides an invaluable resource for every family bookshelf.

ISBN 0 356 17137 X   £5.99 (UK)

IMMUNE POWER: HEALTH AND THE IMMUNE SYSTEM
Jennifer Meek

Our immune system has an amazing capacity to fight illness and disease, but its inefficiency or breakdown can have serious consequences for our health and are related to a variety of conditions, from lacking energy to ME, from recurrent colds to cancer.

This guide shows how you can strengthen your immune system and with a positive attitude enjoy a healthy, active and long life. Written by a qualified nutritional counsellor, it identifies particular diseases and illnesses and covers topics such as diet and nutrition, vitamins and minerals, exercise and sleep, stress and depression, the environment and pollution.

ISBN: 0 356 17138 8   £5.99 (UK)

All Optima books are available at your bookshop or newsagent, or can be ordered from the following address:

Optima, Cash Sales Department,
PO Box 11, Falmouth, Cornwall TR10 9EN

Please send cheque or postal order (no currency), and allow 60p for postage and packing for the first book, plus 25p for the second book and 15p for each additional book ordered up to a maximum charge of £1.90 in the UK.

Customers in Eire and BFPO please allow 60p for the first book, 25p for the second book plus 15p per copy for the next 7 books, thereafter 9p per book.

Overseas customers please allow £1.25 for postage and packing for the first book and 28p per copy for each additional book.